D0013744
W7-BOP-S13

)ITION

Promoting
Wellness
for Prostate Cancer Patients

A GUIDE FOR MEN AND THEIR FAMILIES

Mark A. Moyad, MD, MPH

SpryPublishing
ideas to life

Copyright © 2013 Mark A. Moyad

All rights reserved under International and Pan American Copyright Conventions.

No part of this book may be reproduced or transmitted in any form or by any means electronic or mechanical including photocopying, recording, or by any information storage and retrieval system, without permission in writing from the publisher.

This edition is published by Spry Publishing LLC
2500 South State Street
Ann Arbor, MI 48104 USA

Printed and bound in the United States.

10 9 8 7 6 5 4 3 2 1

Library of Congress Cataloging-in-Publication Data on file.

Paperback ISBN: 978-1-938170-03-4
E-book ISBN: 978-1-938170-07-2
Custom paperback ISBN: 978-1-938170-19-5

Disclaimer: Spry Publishing LLC does not assume responsibility for the contents or opinions expressed herein. Although every precaution is taken to ensure that information is accurate as of the date of publication, differences of opinion exist. The opinions expressed herein are those of the author and do not necessarily reflect the views of the publisher. The information contained in this book is not intended to replace professional advisement of a patient's doctor prior to beginning or changing the patient's course of treatment.

This book is dedicated to my dad and doctor, Robert Moyad.
He taught me what it means to put patients first
and what it means to be a good husband and father.

It is also dedicated to my wife Mia,
who has been my best friend since the day we met.
To say I won the lottery when I met her is actually
an understatement.

And finally, this book is dedicated to the individuals—Epstein,
Jenkins, Pokempner, and Thompson—who invest in the dream
and allow me to make a difference one starfish at a time.

Contents

Introduction

Welcome To The Fourth Edition of *Promoting Wellness for Prostate Cancer Patients: A Guide for Men and Their Families*. This book has been the most widely distributed prostate cancer book in the world for the last 10 years, and it has been translated into multiple languages. It deals with all aspects of prostate cancer—from diet, dietary supplements, and other lifestyle recommendations, to prevention and treatment tips, to managing the common (and not so common) side effects of cancer treatment. Most of the information included in this book is the result of talking to patients, families, and healthcare professionals living and working in all corners of the world. From Alaska to Australia, from Europe to Singapore and South Africa, I find in my travels that we are all spiritually united and so similar in countless ways, including our desire to eliminate cancer from the face of the earth and to have access to the best possible information and care. Therefore, the goal of this fourth edition is the same as all previous ones— to empower you with information and lifestyle suggestions needed to assist you in communicating with your doctor and other healthcare professionals while dealing with prostate cancer. All of the chapters have been updated and expanded and there are added tips, novel reminders, and research to continue to help you increase the chance that you can live a long and overall healthy and happy life. With all of the exciting research underway, I look forward to the day that my book will be placed in a medical museum and no longer needed by a single man. In the meantime, I hope this book and the global movement that is *Promoting Wellness* meet all of your expectations.

All my best,

Mark A. Moyad, MD, MPH
Jenkins/Pokempner Director of
Preventive & Alternative Medicine
University of Michigan Medical Center
Department of Urology
Ann Arbor, Michigan
Email: moyad@umich.edu

Promoting Overall Wellness

When you receive a cancer diagnosis, it may be tempting to focus your wellness activities on the affected area of your body, but there is a basic fact that I'd like you to consider—cardiovascular disease (CVD) is the number one cause of death in men (actually, the leading cause of death for women, too!). Let me repeat this important fact—CVD is the number one cause of death in men—and that includes men diagnosed and treated with prostate cancer!

Prostate cancer treatments are so successful today that, after most men are treated, their risk of dying of prostate cancer becomes somewhat similar to the average man's without prostate cancer risk. So, what is the point of being treated for prostate cancer and not working to reduce your risk of heart disease? In addition, there is now plenty of clinical research to suggest that being heart healthy after being diagnosed with prostate cancer may actually increase the chances of beating prostate cancer itself! Therefore, as we start this section on overall wellness, we will look at some ways that you can reduce your risk of developing heart disease and possibly improve prostate health as well.

Cardiac Health

Know Your Numbers

As we start to explore heart health, we will consider some measurements used to gauge how your body is responding to your lifestyle choices. In the same way that a PSA number or prostate exam provides an initial assessment of your prostate health, knowing your cholesterol and blood pressure numbers can give you a first overview of your cardiac health. A bonus to having your cholesterol regularly measured is that it is a good indicator of how well any lifestyle changes you make are working. In recent dietary studies of individuals with prostate cancer, the individuals who followed the healthiest lifestyle programs also had some of the largest reductions in cholesterol.

So, let's explore what a cholesterol test involves. The blood test is usually done after fasting for 9 to 12 hours and it measures four things—total cholesterol, LDL (bad cholesterol), HDL (good cholesterol), and triglycerides (a type of fat found in your blood). Those items are worth some definition to help you understand their importance.

Total Cholesterol: An overview number developed with a formula applied to LDL, HDL, and triglyceride components. Lower numbers are better unless your HDL is really high.

Low-Density Lipoproteins (LDL): Also called "bad" cholesterol, LDL can cause buildup of plaque on the walls of arteries. The more LDL there is in the blood, the greater the risk of heart disease.

High-Density Lipoproteins (HDL): Also called "good" cholesterol, HDL helps the body get rid of bad cholesterol in the blood. The higher the level of HDL cholesterol, the better. If your levels of HDL are low, your risk of heart disease increases.

Triglycerides: Triglycerides are a type of fat that is carried in the blood. Lower numbers are better.

Cholesterol numbers are measured in mg/dL (milligrams per deciliter) in the United States and mmol/L (millimoles per liter) in other countries. The following table provides information on understanding your cholesterol scores.

Total Cholesterol	
Less than 160 mg/dL (Less than 4.14 mmol/L).	Optimal.
160–200 mg/dL (4.14–5.16 mmol/L).	Desirable.
201–239 mg/dL (5.17–6.19 mmol/L).	Borderline high.
240 mg/dL or higher (6.20 mmol/L or higher).	High.
LDL ("bad cholesterol")	
Less than 70 mg/dL (Less than 1.81 mmol/L).	Ideal for high risk.
Less than 100 mg/dL (Less than 2.59 mmol/L).	Optimal.
100–129 mg/dL (2.59–3.34 mmol/L).	Nearly optimal.
130–159 mg/dL (3.37–4.12 mmol/L).	Borderline high.
160–189 mg/dL (4.14–4.90 mmol/L).	High.
190 mg/dL or higher (4.92 mmol/L or higher).	Very high.
HDL ("good cholesterol")	
60 mg/dL or higher (1.55 mmol/L or higher).	Optimal.
40–59 mg/dL (1.04–1.53 mmol/L).	Normal.
Less than 40 mg/dL (Less than 1.04 mmol/L).	Too low.
Triglycerides ("fat in the blood")	
Less than 150 mg/dL (Less than 1.69 mmol/L).	Normal.
150–199 mg/dL (1.70–2.25 mmol/L).	Borderline high.
200–499 mg/dL (2.26–5.64 mmol/L).	High.
500 mg/dL or higher (5.65 mmol/L or higher).	Very high.

Cholesterol testing is one of the best ways to predict the risk of heart disease. However, it may surprise you to know that almost 50 percent of the men and women who have their first heart attack actually have normal cholesterol numbers! This means that by itself cholesterol testing is not a perfect predictor of cardiac wellness, but it is still the single best blood test routinely available.

In addition to cholesterol screening, there are other blood tests that may improve the evaluation of CVD risk. The hs-CRP blood test (sometimes called the "cardiac CRP" test) probably has the greatest chance of identifying those patients at higher risk of heart disease despite a normal cholesterol level. You should talk to you doctor to see if you should have this test done at the same time that you get a cholesterol blood test. It measures low levels of inflammation that may be occurring, especially in the blood supply around or near the heart. You should not have this test done when you are feeling sick or if you have a bad case of arthritis because that could falsely inflate the test results. Also, do not confuse this test with a basic CRP test (without the letters "hs" in front of it), because the basic CRP test is not as sensitive for predicting heart disease. If your hs-CRP indicates inflammation is an issue, the good news is that many lifestyle changes (good diet, exercise, weight loss) and medications (aspirin, cholesterol-lowering drugs) that reduce cholesterol can also reduce the hs-CRP number.

High-Sensitivity C-Reactive Protein (hs-CRP) Results	
Less than 1 mg/L	Low risk
1–3 mg /L	Moderate risk
Greater than 3 mg/L	High risk

Some medical centers use Apo A and Apo B testing in addition to cholesterol testing. Apo A is a measure of all the heart-protecting (heart-healthy) particles in the blood, and Apo B is a measure of the heart disease–promoting (heart-unhealthy) particles in the blood. Generally speaking, the higher the Apo A number and the lower the Apo B number, the better for your health. The Apo A and B test is used by some doctors to obtain more clarity when the basic cholesterol test results are unclear or when the patient has a history of cardiovascular disease. For example, the Apo testing may be used for patients with fluctuating cholesterol levels or to assess if a patient's consistently low HDL is indeed a serious issue. At times, the ratio of Apo A to Apo B is used as an indicator of health risk similar to the HDL to LDL ratio.

Another number getting a lot of attention these days is your blood glucose (sugar) number. I strongly recommend that everyone get a yearly blood sugar test done. The blood sample is taken when fasting so it can be done at the same time as a cholesterol test. There has been discussion about whether sugar from food feeds cancer, but sugar consumed in food is not a problem as such. In a healthy individual, your body regulates your blood sugar and maintains a stable level to provide energy so that the brain, muscles, and other body areas can survive. However, an uncontrolled blood sugar from prediabetes or diabetes could feed a cancer, as well as damage other body systems. It makes sense to regularly check your blood sugar while doing other heart-healthy blood tests.

Blood Pressure Results	
Less than 120/80 mmHg.	Normal/ low risk.
120–139/80–89 mmHg.	Pre-hypertensive/ moderate risk.
140/90 mmHg or greater.	Hypertensive/ high risk.

In addition to knowing your cholesterol, hs-CRP, and blood sugar numbers, you should have your blood pressure checked regularly. It may be a good idea to purchase your own automated blood pressure machine for use at home. Your local pharmacist can guide you to a reliable machine that is inexpensive. It isn't uncommon for people to experience a falsely elevated blood pressure reading in a doctor's

THE BOTTOM LINE Get your cholesterol, hs-CRP, and blood sugar measured annually (or more often as needed) and discuss your results with your doctor to consider lifestyle changes that can improve your numbers. Monitor your blood pressure regularly. Use the cholesterol and blood pressure goals listed in the previous tables as a guide for discussions with your healthcare professional.

office (called "white coat hypertension"). Taking regular readings will give you a more accurate gauge of your blood pressure than having it checked once or twice a year in the doctor's office. I strongly recommend that everyone buy their own blood pressure device and monitor their blood pressure at least several times a month.

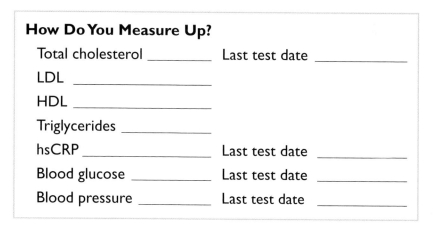

How Do You Measure Up?

Total cholesterol _____ Last test date _____

LDL _____

HDL _____

Triglycerides _____

hsCRP _____ Last test date _____

Blood glucose _____ Last test date _____

Blood pressure _____ Last test date _____

A Healthy Weight

The topic of weight management is never a patient favorite. However, maintaining a healthy weight may be one of the most important things individuals can do, not only to reduce the risk of cancer, but also the progression of the disease. Also, there is no doubt that diet and weight management are central to improving cardiac health. Later in this chapter we'll consider a series of dietary changes that can both improve nutrition and help remove some extra pounds. In a clinical setting, weight is generally tracked by measuring your body mass index (BMI) and waist circumference (WC).

You can figure your BMI using the formula below:

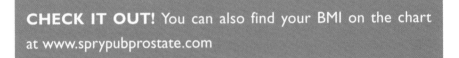

BMI < 25 = Healthy weight

BMI 25 – 29 = Overweight

BMI ≥ 30 = Obese

$$BMI = \frac{lbs.}{inches^2} \times 704$$

$$or = \frac{Kg}{m^2} \left(\frac{weight\ in\ kilograms}{height\ in\ meters^2} \right)$$

(*Note: A BMI comes with one major catch. An individual who has a lot of muscle mass may have a falsely high BMI.*)

CHECK IT OUT! You can also find your BMI on the chart at www.sprypubprostate.com

Physicians may also consider your waist measurement. I'm sure you are wondering why all the concern with waist size? Visceral fat (found deep around the liver, intestines, and stomach) is associated with a greater increase in health problems than subcutaneous fat (just under the skin). Hence, the larger your waist, the greater the risk. If you lose an inch or more of visceral fat, your cholesterol and blood pressure will generally drop almost immediately—a 2-for-1 bonus!

Measure your waist circumference (WC) at your navel. As you might suspect, a high number is a concern. It is desirable to have a WC of 35 inches (89 cm) or less.

We'll look at some specific weight-reduction strategies later in the diet section and you'll find a collection of my favorite diet tips in the appendix at the end of the book. However, in general, I always advise patients to worry most about the calories and not just the fat. Research in the past has focused on lowering your overall fat intake in order to maintain a healthy body weight. Recently this has been challenged (thank goodness!). Today, many dieticians attribute weight struggles to an increasing serving size, and hence an increased calorie count. In other words, more protein, fat, and sugar are contributing to more overweight adults (and children).

To show you what I mean about changing portion size, look at the table relating soda portion sizes and calorie content. This increase in portion size is also seen in everything from burgers to desserts.

Soda Portions		
Decade	Serving size	Total calories
1960s	8 ounces (236 ml)	100 (418 kj)
1970s	12 ounces (354 ml)	150 (628 kj)
1980s	16 ounces (473 ml)	200 (836 kj)
1990s	20 ounces (591 ml)	250 (1046 kj)
2000s	24 ounces (709 ml)	300 (1254 kj)

My favorite mantra is, "Everything in moderation." While you can enjoy your favorite foods, be careful to monitor portion size to control calorie intake and maintain a healthy weight.

How do you measure up?

BMI _____

WC _____

THE BOTTOM LINE Have your BMI and WC measured by your doctor and recorded in your medical chart. The goal is to maintain a normal BMI and WC, or work to reduce your weight so that these numbers move toward a normal range.

Small Steps to Improve Your Diet

Develop a Plan

Every day people make decisions to improve their overall diet plans ... and every day people give up on those plans to improve their diets. Why? In many, many instances it is because they tried to make enormous changes to what they eat all at once. Often their grand diet plans are extreme and require dietary restrictions that leave them feeling deprived of many of their favorite foods. In some cases, the plans restrict even vital nutrients.

When I am advising patients on improving their diet, I urge them to explore numerous dietary plans and pick one with a moderate approach. Overall improvement in diet can be accomplished through a series of smaller changes to improve choices and patients are more likely to stick with several moderate dietary changes than with an extreme, restrictive diet plan.

So what about the low-carb, Mediterranean, low-fat, or Weight Watchers® plans? I suggest that patients talk to their doctor or a nutritionist about these diets, but most depend on lowering your intake of calories and exercising more. Regardless, your primary goal is to maintain a healthy weight, cholesterol, and blood pressure, and one diet or program does not necessarily work for everyone. Programs like Weight Watchers are good because they teach you about food, moderation, and portion sizes. An added benefit is that they also involve a support group. Low carbohydrate diets may work for some individuals, but long-term they can be difficult to follow.

I generally like the Mediterranean diet because it is a moderate and diverse diet with many components. It is flexible, realistic, and practical to follow. A typical Mediterranean diet consists of high monounsaturated and polyunsaturated, and low saturated fat intake, moderate alcohol intake, high consumption of bean products and fiber, cereals, fruits and vegetables, low consumption of meat and meat products, and a moderate intake of milk and dairy products. Basically, this is an "everything in moderation" diet. You'll find that the dietary suggestions that follow align with the principles of the Mediterranean diet plan.

THE BOTTOM LINE Work with your health professional to develop a diet or dietary program that makes sense for you. Keep in mind that if it sounds too good to be true then it probably is. Your health professional should monitor your major indicators; including cholesterol, hs-CRP, blood glucose, blood pressure, weight loss, and PSA level while you are on a new type of diet just to make sure it is working for you.

Eat Primarily Plant-Based Foods

Fruits and Vegetables

Eat a variety of fruits and vegetables and not just tomatoes, pomegranates, or whatever other specific fruit or vegetable du jour is currently getting all of the commercial attention. And don't be overly impressed by the antioxidant amount or value of a single fruit or vegetable. All fruits and vegetables, regardless of their color, have something to offer and their own unique healthy components that add to an overall healthy diet. All fruits and vegetables have some research to suggest they have anti-cancer and, more importantly, anti–heart disease properties.

A warning, be careful to limit fruit and vegetable juices, especially the exotic fruit drinks. You want more antioxidants, but many of these juices are high in calories and price. Some of the so-called healthiest juices are actually unhealthy unless consumed in moderation (less than 8 ounces a day) because they contain too many calories, and they can ultimately contribute to making you obese and unhealthy.

> ## Did you know?
>
> A study was conducted by the National Cancer Institute and involved about 380,000 men and women following a Mediterranean pattern diet. It showed an impact on not just cardiovascular disease but cancer deaths. This dietary pattern has also been associated with lower risks of eye diseases and many others conditions, such as Alzheimer's disease.

Legumes and Seeds

Legumes, such as beans, lentils, and especially soy, and seeds, such as flaxseed and chia seed, are good sources of high-quality protein and they can be used in your diet to replace protein from meat. These products are heart healthy and may reduce your cholesterol. In addition, they are low in saturated and trans fat, high in fiber, and just overall prostate healthy. The Food and Drug Administration (FDA) suggests that 25 grams a day of soy protein from a variety of traditional sources may reduce the risk of heart disease along with a reduction in saturated fat intake.

DR. MOYAD'S FAST FAVES Drink Selections Under 100 Calories	
Beverage	**Calories (8 oz. serving)**
Skim milk	90 (377 kj)
Soy milk	90 (377 kj)
Carrot juice	75 (314 kj)
Almond milk	40 (167 kj)
Coffee or tea	5 (21 kj)
Diet soda (with caffeine)	0
Water	0

Like soy products, flaxseed can be a great tasting and healthy addition to your diet. Whole or ground flaxseed may be purchased in the vitamin/supplement department of most retailers carrying these types of products. You can grind the whole seeds or purchase containers of ground flaxseed. Like most foods that are high in fiber, too much (more than a few tablespoons a day) can be upsetting to your system.

DR. MOYAD'S FAST FAVES Healthiest Soy Products		
Product	**Serving**	**Total Protein**
Soybean (Edamame)	I cup	20 grams
Tempeh	½ cup	20 grams
Tofu	I cup	20 grams
Soy protein powder	I scoop	15 grams
Soy milk	I cup	10 grams

Whole Grains

By definition, a whole grain product is one that contains all the essential parts and naturally-occurring nutrients of the entire grain seed. If the grain has been processed (e.g., cracked, crushed, rolled, extruded, and/or cooked), the food product should deliver approximately the same rich balance of nutrients that are found in the original grain seed to be considered "whole grain." Both nutritious and high in fiber, whole grain products have been shown to be a good choice in a healthy diet.

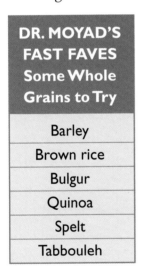

DR. MOYAD'S FAST FAVES Some Whole Grains to Try
Barley
Brown rice
Bulgur
Quinoa
Spelt
Tabbouleh

Did you know?

Recently, the American Society for Nutrition brought together researchers to review the evidence regarding the health benefits associated with whole grains. Current scientific evidence indicates that whole grains play an important role in lowering the risk of chronic diseases, such as coronary heart disease, diabetes, and cancer, and also contribute to body weight management and gastrointestinal health.

Nuts in Your Diet

Most nuts are high in vitamins and minerals, high in other antioxidants, low in saturated fat, high in monounsaturated fat, and some even contain omega-3 fatty acids. Also, nuts as a snack give you a sense of being full without getting too many calories. It is interesting that nuts such as walnuts, almonds, pistachios, Brazil nuts, and others have been associated with a lower risk of sudden cardiac death, and they contain compounds associated with prostate health.

THE BOTTOM LINE Consider making plant-based foods, such as fruits, vegetables, legumes, seeds, whole grains, and nuts, the base for your healthy diet plan. By experimenting and trying some new selections, you are sure to find some new personal favorites.

DR. MOYAD'S FAST FAVES—Some Nuts and Seeds

(Serving = 1 ounce or 1/4 cup = 150–200 calories)	Nutrition
Almonds (170 calories/771 kj)	High in monounsaturated fat (10 g). Polyunsaturated fat (4 g). Saturated fat (1 g). High in potassium (210 mg), fiber (3 g), and vitamin E.
Brazil nuts (190 calories/795 kj)	Monounsaturated fat (7 g). Polyunsaturated fat (21 g). Saturated fat (4 g). High in potassium (190 mg). High in selenium (6–8 times the recommended daily allowance).
Cashews (160 calories/669 kj)	High in monounsaturated fat (8 g). Potassium (160 mg).
Chestnuts (50–100 calories/ 209-419 kj per 3 roasted nuts)	Equal amounts of monounsaturated (0.1 g), polyunsaturated (0.1 g), and saturated fat (0.1 g). Lowest in calories and fat, and high in water content. High in potassium (600 mg) and fiber (1.5 g). Only nut with a lot of vitamin C (about 10 mg).
Hazelnuts/filberts (180 calories/753 kj)	High in monounsaturated fat (13 g). High in potassium (210 mg) and fiber (3 g).

DR. MOYAD'S FAST FAVES—Some Nuts and Seeds	
(Serving = 1 ounce or 1/4 cup = 150–200 calories)	Nutrition
Macadamia (200 calories/838 kj)	Monounsaturated fat (17 g). Polyunsaturated fat (0 g).
Peanuts (170 calories/711 kj)	Higher in monounsaturated (7 g) than polyunsaturated fat (4 g). High in potassium (190 mg). High in resveratrol (anti-aging compound?).
Pecans (200 calories/838 kj)	High in monounsaturated fat (12 g). High in fiber (3 g).
Pine nuts (190 calories/795 kj)	High in polyunsaturated fat (10g). High in potassium (170 mg).
Pistachios (160 calories/669 kj)	High in monounsaturated fat (7 g). High in potassium (300 mg) and fiber (3 g).
Sesame seeds (200 calories/838 kj)	Almost equal amounts of monounsaturated and polyunsaturated fats. High in healthy plant estrogen. High in calcium (350 mg), iron (5 mg), magnesium (125 mg), potassium (170 mg), and fiber (4 g).
Soy nuts (150 calories/628 kj)	High in polyunsaturated fat (2 times more) compared to monounsaturated fat. High in potassium (325 mg) and fiber (4 g).

DR. MOYAD'S FAST FAVES—Some Nuts and Seeds (Serving = 1 ounce or 1/4 cup = 150–200 calories)	Nutrition
Sunflower seeds (170 calories/711 kj)	High in polyunsaturated fat (9g). High in potassium (240 mg) and fiber (3 g).
Walnuts (190 calories/795 kj)	High in omega-3 polyunsaturated fat (13 g). Highest nut source of plant omega-3 (ALA).

Eat More Healthy Fats and Oils

In addition to considering your overall calorie count, you should also consider the types of fat you are consuming. The following table gives you an overview of common dietary fats and their effects on your body.

There are two types of fat that you should be concerned about—saturated fat, also known as "hydrogenated fat," and trans fat, also known as "partially hydrogenated fat." High intake of these types of fat has been linked to heart disease and cancer. Choosing some of the more healthy fats, such as monounsaturated and polyunsaturated fats, is not only heart healthy, but also seems prostate healthy. A recent study showed that men consuming lower amounts of saturated fats and calories also had a lower risk of prostate cancer returning after treatment.

Type of Dietary Fat	Where Is It Commonly Found?	Good or Bad Fat & Impact on Cholesterol
Monounsaturated fat	Healthy plant-based cooking oils (canola, olive), nuts.	Good. Lowers LDL & increases HDL.
Polyunsaturated fat (includes omega-3 fatty acids)	Healthy plant-based cooking oils (canola, safflower, soybean), flaxseed, fish, nuts, soybeans.	Good. Lowers LDL & increases HDL.
Saturated fat (also known as hydrogenated fat)	Non-lean meat, high-fat dairy, some fast foods.	Some are bad. Increases LDL & increases HDL (note how it increases HDL ... interesting, isn't it?).
Trans fat (also known as partially hydrogenated fat)	Some margarine, fast foods, snack foods, deep-fried foods.	Bad. Increases LDL & lowers HDL.

Cooking oils that are high in monounsaturated fat, high in omega-3 fatty acids, and lower in saturated and trans fat are not only heart healthy but also may be prostate

> **!** Replace butter with a healthy oil, such as olive oil, in cooking or for dipping pieces of bread.

healthy. Oils such as soybean, canola, olive, and safflower are just some of the healthy oils out there. Do not just focus on

Did you know?

One of the largest government-funded studies in the history of medicine was called the DASH (Dietary Approaches to Stop Hypertension) study. The great thing about this original study was that it involved pre-hypertensive people not taking prescription medications. Half of the participants were women and 60 percent were African-Americans. In analyzing results of this study, it was amazing to find that eating healthy and lowering sodium intake had a wonderfully positive impact on blood pressure numbers. Currently, it is recommended that a healthy individual gets not more than 2,300 milligrams of sodium (1 teaspoon) per day but, in the DASH diet, the effective dose was 1,500 milligrams of sodium per day. (Many people are regularly consuming 3,500 to 4,500 milligrams per day!) The DASH participants experienced an average drop in blood pressure of 11 mmHg systolic and 6 mmHg diastolic—a drop this large is generally obtained by using blood pressure–reducing medications.

olive oil, because numerous oils are beneficial. However, be careful of the amount used because 1 tablespoon of any oil contains approximately 120 calories/502 kj (everything in moderation)!

Reduce Total Salt Consumption

Since about 80 percent of your daily sodium intake comes from processed foods and only about 5 percent from the saltshaker, it is very important to carefully check the sodium content on nutritional labels. Don't be fooled by products marked "lower sodium." A quick look at some average sodium contents below gives you an idea of how much they may vary for a particular product. Read your labels carefully!

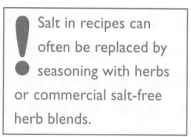 Salt in recipes can often be replaced by seasoning with herbs or commercial salt-free herb blends.

- Breads 100 to 200 mg of sodium in 1 slice
- Chicken with rice soup (condensed) 600 to 1,300 mg of sodium in 1/2 cup
- Frozen pizza (plain) 400 to 1,200 mg of sodium in 4 ounces
- Frozen vegetables 5 to 150 mg of sodium in 1/2 cup
- Potato chips 100 to 200 mg of sodium in 1 ounce
- Pretzels 250 to 600 mg of sodium in 1 ounce
- Salad dressing (regular) 50 to 250 mg of sodium in 1 tablespoon
- Salsa 75 to 150 mg of sodium in 1 tablespoon

- Soda 10 to 100 mg of sodium in 8 ounces
- Tomato juice 350 to 1,000 mg of sodium in 8 ounces
- Tomato soup 600 to 1,300 mg of sodium in 1/2 cup

THE BOTTOM LINE Read labels carefully to reduce the amount of sodium you are consuming in packaged foods.

Limit Red Meat and Increase Fish and Poultry

In a traditional Mediterranean Diet plan, little red meat is consumed and fish and poultry are eaten more regularly. Several times a month when red meat is part of a meal, lean cuts are used and the portion is limited to around the size of a deck of cards. Sausage, bacon, and other high fat red meats should be mostly avoided.

Adding fish to your diet several days a week can be a delicious way to reduce your consumption of red meat and

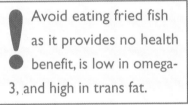 Avoid eating fried fish as it provides no health benefit, is low in omega-3, and high in trans fat.

boost your consumption of omega-3 fatty acids at the same time. Omega-3 fatty acids, especially from fish, are not only heart healthy but, you guessed it, they are also prostate healthy. One of the largest medical studies of fish consumption found that eating fish several times a week was associated with a lower risk of advanced or aggressive prostate cancer. Some recent research suggests a lower risk of cancer recurrence after conventional treatment when fish intake was increased.

However, there has been a recent concern that some large fish (king mackerel, shark, swordfish, and tilefish) contain high concentrations of mercury, which can be bad for your health. This concern is generally important for women who are pregnant or trying to get pregnant and young children.

DR. MOYAD'S FAST FAVES Fish with Highest Total Omega-3 Content	
Salmon	1,775 mg
Herring	1,710 mg
Great Lakes Whitefish	1,350 mg
Anchovy	1,165 mg
Mackerel (Atlantic)	1,060 mg
Trout	800 mg

Both wild fish and farmed fish are good sources of omega-3. Farmed fish are fed products that contain fish protein and fish oil. Wild fish actually have a slightly more unpredictable amount of omega-3 because the amount depends on the maturity of the fish and when it is caught. It should be kept in mind that the positives still outweigh the negatives for farmed fish. Overall, the amount of contaminants in farmed fish is usually low, and it is still better to eat these fish than to not eat fish at all.

Recent studies of farm-raised fish (such as salmon) have shown that they can contain as much as 50 to 75 percent less vitamin D compared to wild fish. Some farm-raised salmon also have vitamin D2, whereas the more natural vitamin D3 is found in wild salmon. The cause of this difference requires further investigation, but farm-raised fish is still considered healthy to eat.

CHECK IT OUT! Visit www.sprypubprostate.com for a chart of the omega-3 content of your favorite fish.

Consume More Fiber

Many foods contain a high amount of fiber—beans, fruits, vegetables, bran cereals, flaxseed, chia seeds, whole grains, and oats, to name a few. These products not only lower cholesterol but they also seem to reduce your risk of a variety of problems and may even be immune healthy. Keep in mind that if you increase your intake of fiber, you should also increase your consumption of water.

Some benefits of increasing fiber consumption are:

- Helps with weight control because it delays the emptying of stomach contents, delays the absorption of fats, and promotes a feeling of fullness.
- Improves glucose or sugar balance by delaying the movement and absorption of carbohydrates into the small intestine, so you simply burn your dietary fuel more efficiently and evenly.
- Reduces cholesterol levels by binding with cholesterol-carrying products in the intestine and causing it to be excreted or eliminated.
- Reduces the colon transit time and pressure within the colon.
- Reduces the risk of a number of digestive conditions—diverticulitis, irritable bowel syndrome (IBS), hemorrhoids, and gastroesophageal reflux disease (GERD)—and promotes increases in healthy bacteria in the colon to improve overall digestive health.
- Reduces blood pressure and may reduce a man's PSA blood test number by lowering cholesterol.

Most fiber dietary supplements and powders contain only soluble fiber, which can create too much bloating and gas and you may have to take up to 50 pills a day to get your daily intake of fiber. You can get additional fiber from some fruits and vegetables, bean products, nuts and seeds, whole grains, and even fiber bars. However, look for the fiber bar that is lowest in calories, sodium, and unhealthy fats and highest in insoluble fiber. Mostly insoluble fiber is better because, unlike soluble fiber, it does not cause excess gas production in the bowel but still gives you the benefits of fiber.

> **!** The simplest way to boost your fiber intake is to eat a cereal in the morning and add flaxseed, chia seeds, small fruits, or other simple fiber sources (oat bran) to it. For example, bran cereal provides 13 to 15 grams of fiber per 1/3 cup (much smaller than a bowl of cereal). Add several tablespoons of flaxseed or chia seed and you have almost 20 grams of fiber in one meal. You have almost reached your daily requirement in just one serving of cereal!

Read Those Labels Carefully

When you are making changes to your diet, it is important that you read nutritional labels carefully. You will see many advertising claims on packaged food—LOWER SODIUM! REDUCED CALORIES! LOW FAT! LITE!—but, what exactly do those claims really mean? The only way to know for sure is by reading the nutritional labels. But, what are you looking for there?

Is this cholesterol-lowering margarine a healthy product? YES! It is low in calories, high in healthy types of fat (poly- and monoun- saturated) and low in the un- healthy types of fat (satu- rated and trans fat). It is also low in choles- terol, sodium, carbohydrates, and protein, which is why it is also low in calories.

Nutrition Facts Serving Size = I Tbsp.	
Calories 70 (293 kj)	Cholest. 0 mg
Fat Calories 70 (293 kj)	Sodium 110 mg
Total Fat 8 g	Total Carb. 0 g
Sat. Fat 1 g	Protein 0 g
Trans Fat 0 g	
Polyunsat. Fat 2 g	
Monounsat. Fat 4.5 g	

When you visit the grocery store, don't blindly pick up the brand that you usually purchase. Take a minute to look over the nutritional information and then pick up other prod- ucts in the section to compare nutritional information. Chal- lenge yourself to check out a couple of food choices every time you visit the store and try at least one new product each week. You may find that you really enjoy foods that are nu- tritionally better choices.

Remember, as we discussed earlier, improving your diet can be accomplished by making many small measured steps. You don't have to give up all your favorite foods, but you might look at the nutritional label and decide to make a food a special monthly treat as opposed to a weekly staple. Small steps, big results!

A Word About Alcohol

All types of alcohol (beer, hard liquor, red wine, and white wine) in moderation may be healthy, but in excess all types of alcohol are unhealthy. Red wine has never been proven to be healthier than any other type of alcoholic drink, and all forms of alcohol are equally dangerous in excess.

Let's review a "serving" of alcohol:
- One serving of beer = 12 ounces /354 ml (about 13.2 grams of alcohol)
- One serving of hard liquor = 1.5 ounce/44 ml shot of 80 proof liquor (15.1 grams of alcohol)
- One serving of wine = 4–6 ounces/118-177 ml (about 10.8 to 15 grams of alcohol)
- 1 gram of alcohol = about 7 calories/29 kj.

Now, it is important to understand what is meant by "moderate amounts of alcohol"—for women one serving a day, and for men, one to two servings of alcohol per day.

Consider what alcohol in moderation may do for you:
- Increase good cholesterol or HDL
- Reduce your risk of a heart attack or stroke (may thin your blood or reduce stickiness of clot-forming platelets, reduce fibrinogen)
- Improve mental health

- May improve prostate health and sexual function (controversial)

Alcohol in excess can cause many problems, including:
- Increases triglycerides
- Increases sugar levels
- Increases the risk of osteoporosis
- Large source of calories (weight gain)
- Increases blood pressure
- Damages the heart
- Suppresses the immune system
- Reduces the amount of healthy nutrients found in the blood
- Increases the risk of some cancers—oral/esophageal and breast cancer and possibly many other cancers such as lung cancer
- Increases histamine levels and may make allergies worse
- Reduces sexual performance

Get Moving!

What if I told you that you could take a magical, low-cost, safe pill that would reduce the risk of developing or slow the progression of some of the most serious health conditions? Would you take it? Sure you would! Suppose I told you

> ! Research has shown that regular exercise can reduce both the risk and recurrence of depression.

that the magical pill was 30 minutes of exercise (your choice of activity) every day? Are you surprised to find that there are so many beneficial results of exercising?

Exercise comes in a variety of forms and you should pick the one that works for you long term. Some people like to walk or climb stairs; others like to swim, row, or use a treadmill or elliptical machine; and others still like to garden. Basically, the amount of physical activity you should do and the frequency of the activity are dependent on your weight. An individual should do enough exercise to help himself maintain a healthy weight. Obviously though, the more active you are the better.

Exercise intensity is often measured using a metabolic equivalent task (MET) score. A single MET is the energy that is expended by just sitting quietly. MET scores are used by some researchers to calculate the average intensity of a specific exercise. MET scores for specific exercises are defined as the ratio of the metabolic rate associated with a specific

Did you know?

Studies have shown that people who exercise regularly have a 25 to 50 percent reduction in the occurrence of many potentially serious diseases, including heart disease, osteoporosis, Alzheimer's disease, colon cancer, stroke, and type II diabetes. Also, in a recent study of men in the United States, those exercising almost every day were found to have a greater chance of surviving prostate cancer.

DR. MOYAD'S FAST FAVES		
Weight-Lifting Exercises		
Weight-Lifting Exercise	**Initial Repetition**	**Additional Repetition**
Biceps curl	12 to 15	8 to 10
Chest press	12 to 15	8 to 10
Latissimus pull-down	12 to 15	8 to 10
Modified curl-ups	12 to 15	8 to 10
Overhead press	12 to 15	8 to 10
Triceps extension	12 to 15	8 to 10
Calf raises	12 to 15	8 to 10
Leg curl	12 to 15	8 to 10
Leg extension	12 to 15	8 to 10
Spine bone building exercise*	8 to 12 modified push-ups	8 to 12 modified push-ups

*Some doctors or trainers also like to include a back lift in order to strengthen the spine. A small weight (just a few pounds or kilograms), usually in the form of a cushion or bean bag, is placed on the upper back between the shoulder blades. While lying on your stomach, do 8 to 12 modified push-ups (stomach stays on the floor, hands clasped together behind your head, and lift your upper body up then down, up and down). This places resistance on the spine and may improve bone mineral density in this area.

activity divided by the resting metabolic rate. For example, if someone walks at an average pace, they are generally assigned a MET score of 3; jogging, a MET score of 7; and running, a MET score of 12. The higher the number of METs during your exercise routine, the greater the workout for your heart. You will see this principle in action the next time you get on an exercise machine that reports METs.

Also, keep in mind that weight lifting is probably as important as regular aerobic exercise. Weight lifting just a 2 to 3 times a week for 20 to 30 minutes lowers your risk of osteoporosis, lowers your risk of type II diabetes, helps you to maintain a healthy weight, reduces the risk of heart disease, increases energy levels, and may improve your quality of life. Talk with your doctor to see which exercises might be most appropriate for your situation. By starting slowly and sticking with an exercise plan, you may be surprised how many health benefits you experience!

THE BOTTOM LINE Take your exercise pill every day! Pick exercises that you enjoy. The amount of time you exercise should depend on your weight—whatever it takes to maintain a healthy weight is best. Begin to give weight lifting the same importance as aerobic exercise. Start to exercise in moderation. Exercising beyond your capability may result in injury and suppressing of your immune system.

As we wrap up the heart health and diet sections, let's take a minute to see how healthy your lifestyle choices are and set some personal goals. I use this checklist whenever I speak to patient groups and healthcare workers. The research behind the test came from studies conducted in over 50 countries around the world, including both men and women of all races, ages, and professions. See how your lifestyle stacks up. If you answer no to a question, consider a health improvement goal to enter.

Healthy Personal Lifestyle Questions

Score one point for every time you answer yes.

1. I do NOT currently smoke cigarettes/cigars or use any tobacco products (chewing tobacco).

_____ Yes, I agree with the statement.

What goal might improve your health and score?

_____

_____

_____

2. I have regular cholesterol screenings done and have a normal level and a normal hs-CRP test. (Check pages 11–13 for normal levels.)

_____ Yes, I agree with the statement.

What goal might improve your health and score?

_____

_____

_____

3. I have my blood pressure checked regularly and have a normal pressure. (Check page 14 for normal levels.)

_____ Yes, I agree with the statement.

What goal might improve your health and score?

_____

_____

_____

4. I have a normal blood glucose level and have NOT been diagnosed with diabetes.

_____ Yes, I agree with the statement.

What goal might improve your health and score?

_____

_____

_____

_____

5. I have a normal (not overweight or obese) waist circumference.

_____ Yes, I agree with the statement.

What goal might improve your health and score?

_____

_____

_____

_____

6. I do not currently have depression, high stress, or other mental health issues.

_____ Yes, I agree with the statement.

What goal might improve your health and score?

_____

_____

_____

_____

7. I eat several servings of fruits and vegetables per day.

_____ Yes, I agree with the statement.

What goal might improve your health and score?

_____

_____

_____

_____

8. I drink alcohol in moderation or not at all. (1 drink a day maximum for women and 1–2 maximum for men)

_____ Yes, I agree with the statement.

What goal might improve your health and score?

_____

_____

_____

_____

9. I do at least 30 minutes of aerobic exercise per day on average.

_____ Yes, I agree with the statement.

What goal might improve your health and score?

_____

_____

_____

_____

10. I lift weights or do some type of resistance exercise at least 2–3 times per week.

_____ Yes, I agree with the statement.

What goal might improve your health and score?

_____

_____

_____

_____

Total Score _____

What does my score mean?

10 points =	Congratulations!
7-9 points =	Very Good! Keep up the good work and 10 points is within your reach!
4-6 points =	Good! However, still a lot to work on.
1-3 points =	Okay! Still need to make some major life changes very soon.
0 points =	Need to change things now!

What does my score really mean in terms of health?

Men and women who lived the longest had the highest number of moderate healthy lifestyle choices. If someone had almost 10, or all 10, "yes" answers, there was about a 70 percent chance that they would live to at least age 85 without mental or physical disability. Each positive lifestyle choice gave the individual a 5–10% decreased risk of dying young or suffering from a cardiovascular event (heart attack, for example). The more of the lifestyle changes that you are able to accomplish, the greater the chance that you will not only live a longer life, but a more high-quality life! Finally, keep in mind that if you have any of the above conditions (such as depression, elevated glucose, or high cholesterol levels), but they are currently under medical and lifestyle control, then you can change your answer to "yes."

Dietary Checklist

See how you stack up against the participants in the National Cancer Institute study of men and women following a Mediterranean diet plan. Individuals with scores of 6 or more on the checklist begin to see a lower risk of dying young as compared to those with scores of 4 or less. More dietary tips can be found in Appendix One.

Beverage or Food	Your Score. Add one point for each yes answer		
Alcohol—1/2 to 1 drink for women, 1 to 2 for men (but no more).	Yes	No	
Fat intake focused on healthy fats, mostly monounsaturated and polyunsaturated fats (canola, olive, safflower oil, etc.).	Yes	No	
Fish—4 or more servings per week.	Yes	No	
Fruit—3 or more servings a day.	Yes	No	
Legumes/beans—2 or more servings per week.	Yes	No	
Red and processed meat—1 or fewer servings per day.	Yes	No	
Nuts and seeds—2 or more servings per week.	Yes	No	
Vegetables (other than potatoes)—4 or more servings a day.	Yes	No	
Whole grains—2 or more servings a day.	Yes	No	
Total Score	Points		

Note: I have not specified which types of each food are best for your health but you'll find some tips in Appendix One. Traditional Mediterranean diets also allow moderate intake of dairy, such as cheese, milk, and yogurt. Healthy, non-processed foods with more fiber and protein are encouraged.

References:

"INTERHEART Study." Lancet 2004; 364: 937–952.

"Framingham Heart Study." Journal of American Geriatric Society 2005; 53: 1944–1950.

"INTERHEART Study." Journal of American Medical Association 2007; 297: 286–94.

"Honolulu Heart Program & Asia Aging Study." Journal of American Medical Association 2006; 296: 2343–50.

"Physicians' Health Study." Arch Internal Medicine 2008; 168: 284–90.

"Genetic Risk Score versus Traditional Risk Factors Study" Journal of American Medical Association 2010; 303: 631-637.

"National Cancer Institute, www.cancer.gov"

"Mediterranean Diet Study & All-Cause Mortality." Mitrou PN, et al. Arch Internal Medicine 2007; 167: 2461–2468.

"National Health and Nutrition Examination Survey (NHANES)" Journal of the American Medical Association 2012; 307: 1273-1283.

Dietary Supplements

Now that you have taken steps to make heart- and prostate-healthy lifestyle changes, you are ready to consider what supplements may be of value to you. We've attempted to provide general information on some of the most common ones considered of use to prostate cancer patients. This information should give you a starting point for discussions with your healthcare provider on which of the practices would be good choices for your personal situation. You should always consult with your doctor before starting to take a particular supplement.

When it comes to any dietary supplement, I believe less is more and megadoses are never better. Every individual supplement that I have ever researched comes with serious side effects when taken in large doses beyond what is truly needed. In fact, many megadose supplement studies suggest a worse outcome or prognosis in patients with cancer. In other words, talk to your doctor about whether or not you actually qualify for any pill or supplement based on your medical history and from the results of your latest medical tests. If you do qualify, talk to your doctor about the precise dose, frequency, and form or brand name of the supplement that was used in the best objective clinical studies that suggested a benefit. This is exactly the same standard doctors use for prescription medications and dietary supplements should be treated in the same manner.

Aspirin

Low-dose aspirin (81 to 100 milligrams) continues to be one of the most promising over-the-counter products (OTCs) to reduce the risk of cardiovascular disease (heart attack and ischemic stroke, for example) in high-risk individuals. There is some human research to suggest that aspirin may reduce the risk and progression of several cancers, including colon and even prostate cancer. However, many people take aspirin without truly qualifying for this medication and, in that case, the risk of side effects may outweigh the benefits. Never just start taking aspirin to prevent or treat cancer or even heart disease without talking to your doctor. I like to see at least some type of risk-to-benefit calculation, such as a Framingham Risk Score, completed before starting aspirin treatment. Men who do NOT have an increased risk for ulcers and/or internal bleeding, normal or low blood pressure (with or without medication), and have a 10-year risk of a cardiovascular event that is around 10 percent or higher (from the Framingham or Reynolds risk score) are potential candidates.

Regular or daily use of non-steroidal anti-inflammatory drugs (NSAIDs), such as ibuprofen or Motrin®, or prescription COX-2 inhibitor drugs such as Celebrex® and others, should NOT be used for prostate cancer prevention or treatment unless approved by the primary care doctor or cardiologist, because the risk of side effects is generally greater than the benefits they can provide for you.

> **!** Check out your Framingham Risk Score by visiting the American Heart Association website, www.americanheart.org, or www.reynoldsriskscore.org for more information.

B-Vitamin Dietary Supplements
(including B1, B2, B3, B6, B12, and Folic Acid)

Over the past 10 years, numerous clinical trials were started in the hope of finding that high doses of B vitamins could reduce the risk of cardiovascular disease and even cancer. However, researchers have been surprised to learn that megadose B vitamins may actually promote heart disease and encourage the growth of cancer. Many cancers, including prostate cancer, have receptors for large doses of B vitamins, especially folic acid. In other words, researchers believe that these tumors may use certain vitamins as nutrients to help them grow. The large clinical trials have suggested that "less is more" when it comes to considering vitamins and minerals.

The only B vitamin that needs to be taken in higher doses by some individuals with heart disease is vitamin B3, which is also known as niacin. This B vitamin can increase HDL and lower LDL and triglycerides and it can be used with a statin drug. Niacin comes in a prescription or an over-the-counter version. It is heart healthy, but does come with side effects, which is why only some individuals qualify for it.

On rare occasions, some people may also qualify for slightly higher doses of B12 or folic acid because their blood level is so low that it can cause problems with their health. Regardless, most individuals reading this book need to just stick to healthy food and a children's multivitamin once daily to get their recommended daily allowance of B vitamins.

DR. MOYAD'S FAST FAVES Dietary Sources of B Vitamins
Beans
Bananas
Potatoes
Tuna
Turkey
Whole grains

Calcium and Vitamin D

Since they relate to each other so closely and both are

crucial to bone health, we'll consider them together. Calcium, vitamin D, and weight lifting do reduce bone fractures as long as you can take your dietary supplement pills (about 80 percent of the time) and exercise regularly. Bone health is not only an issue with some testosterone-reducing treatments for prostate cancer, but it is fast becoming a serious concern for men in general as they get older.

Let's review the approximate requirements for total calcium (mg) and vitamin D (IU-international units) daily intake, combining diet and supplements.

Age	Calcium (mg)	Vitamin D
19–49 years	1,000	600 IU (15 mcg)
50–70 years	1,000	600 IU (15 mcg)
Over 70 years	1,200	800 IU (20 mcg)

Institute of Medicine (IOM) and Dietary Reference Intakes for Calcium and Vitamin D (www.iom.edu/vitamind)

As you can see from the chart, men generally need a daily total of calcium of 1,000 to 1,200 milligrams from foods, beverages, and/or supplements. After you are able to determine your dietary calcium intake, you may find you need more from food sources or dietary supplements. Calcium supplements are effective at reducing the risk of fractures, however, if they are not taken regularly (about 24–25 days of every month), they simply do not work in many cases. Your doctor and/or nutritionist should determine the specific amount of calcium needed based on your individual needs. There has been some concern lately that getting too much calcium from supplements may increase the risk of cardiovascular disease. For this reason it is critical to determine your calcium intake from foods or beverages before deciding on using supplemental calcium.

Ideally, calcium dietary supplements should be taken in divided doses throughout the day, because the human body generally absorbs approximately 500 mg of elemental calcium at a time. If you take more than this at once, you will not absorb as much as if you spread the dosages out. Some of the supplements may also contain vitamin D, which increases capsule/tablet size just a little.

DR. MOYAD'S FAST FAVES Foods Rich in Calcium	
Collard greens	360 mg
Orange juice (fortified)	350 mg
Sardines	325 mg
Oatmeal	325 mg
Yogurt	300 mg
Milk	300 mg
Cheese	275 mg

Let's spend a bit more time on vitamin D. It is important to consider one blood test that can be expensive (check with your insurance company) but may tell you and your doctor about your risk of a future fracture. This is the vitamin D blood test. Normal blood levels of vitamin D are needed to maintain proper bone health. The 25-hydroxy-vitamin D (25-OH vitamin D) test is the preferred test for most patients, but a second test may also be used in patients with abnormal kidney function. Experts agree that normal results

Type of Calcium Supplement	Elemental Calcium by Weight	Comments
Calcium carbonate	40%	Most tested; requires fewest pills/day; can be used as an acid reflux drug. Least expensive. Should be taken with food because you need some stomach acid to absorb these supplements, in general. May slightly increase the risk of constipation and kidney stones.
Calcium citrate or Calcium citrate malate	21%	Best choice for those with a history of kidney stones, better absorbed, especially in a low-acid stomach environment so it can be taken with with or without food. More expensive & more pills needed daily, so longterm compliance can be an issue.
Calcium phosphate	38% or 31%	Fewer pills to take, in general. Tricalcium or dicalcium phosphate. Can be taken with or without food. Simplicity and price getting closer to calcium carbonate. Need many more clinical trials before they will be recommended on a regular basis.

for a 25-OH vitamin D test are approximately 30–40 ng/ml or 75–100 nmol/L. Some tests may run a little higher or lower, but this is a good goal for men concerned about bone loss. Some advocates are calling for really high vitamin D blood levels, for example 60 ng/ml (150 nmol/L) or higher, but I do not support this recommendation. I have never seen a situation where more is indeed better when there is no good human research to support the belief.

Regardless, what all of this means is that most people would need to take about 800 to 1,000 IU (or more) just to achieve a normal blood level of vitamin D. I suggest that you let the 25-OH vitamin D test result and your doctor's advice help you to decide how much vitamin D you need to take daily. Keep in mind that the test is most accurate when it is done in the late fall or wintertime, because this is when vitamin D levels tend to be the lowest (due to less ultraviolet B-light exposure from the sun). However, if necessary, the test can be done any time of the year.

If your blood test results suggest that you need more vitamin D, it can be obtained from the following sources:

- Fortified beverages and foods—milk, soy, protein bars, and cereal. Only eggs, mushrooms, and seafood contain vitamin D naturally, but varieties of other beverages and foods are fortified with vitamin D. Check the label on the product to determine the amount.
- Fish and fish oils—Fish and some fish oil supplements contain a high level of vitamin D.

- Sun (ultraviolet B light) 10–15 minutes of sunlight several times per week, especially during the spring and summer, allows the human body to make some vitamin D. Sunscreen users, African Americans, overweight, and older individuals have a more difficult time making this vitamin.
- Children's multivitamin or an individual vitamin D supplement—most contain at least 400 IU of vitamin D.
- Prescription drugs—Calcitriol and other vitamin D sources can be prescribed and taken orally or given as an injection if the doctor thinks you need to get vitamin D from these sources.

Keep in mind that, in general, 100 IU (2.5 mcg) of vitamin D per day is needed just to raise your blood level about 1 ng/ml (2.5 nmol/L) after 2–3 months. So, if you need to raise your blood level 4 ng/ml (10 nmol/L) you would need to take 400 IU (10 mcg) of vitamin D per day. If you need to raise your level 10 ng/ml (25 nmol/L), you guessed it, you would need 1,000 IU (25 mcg) of vitamin D per day for 2–3 months. The bottom line is that after you normalize your vitamin D blood test, 800 to 1,000 IU of vitamin D per day should help to maintain it unless directed otherwise by your doctor based on blood test results.

DR. MOYAD'S FAST FAVES Fish Rich in Vitamin D		
Salmon (wild)	1,000 IU	(25 mcg)
Oysters	545 IU	(14 mcg)
Catfish	425 IU	(11 mcg)
Bluefish	415 IU	(10 mcg)
Mackerel	395 IU	(10 mcg)

There are basically two types of vitamin D supplements available for over-the-counter purchase—vitamin D2 (also known as "ergocalciferol") and vitamin D3 (also known as "cholecalciferol"). Vitamin D3 is the type that most experts believe should be taken if you have a choice. Some of the many reasons vitamin D3 is preferred are: vitamin D3 is the form that humans make naturally from sunlight and the type found in wild fish; it is just as cost effective as vitamin D2 and raises the long term blood test results better than D2, and vitamin D3 has been used in most of the human studies to prevent bone loss in men and women. However, vegans should use vitamin D2 dietary supplements because they come from plant sources and vitamin D3 supplements usually come from animal sources.

Whether or not you should take calcium and vitamin D supplements is dependent on whether or not you qualify for these pills. Tallying dietary intake or, in the case of vitamin D, measuring your blood level with a blood test can determine if you need to supplement either calcium or vitamin D. Discuss bone health and these two supplements with your doctor to figure out what is best for your individual situation.

Fiber-Based Dietary Supplements
Although discussed briefly earlier in the chapter, I thought they were worth considering here as well. There is little need to spend money on fiber pills because you would need large numbers of pills each day to reach the recommended daily allowance for fiber. Save your money. Fiber powders, wafers,

and crackers can be expensive and most contain the type of fiber that can cause a lot of gas and bloating. Fiber-based or bran and oatmeal-based cereal or porridge with ground flaxseed or chia seed on top is a good way to get your fiber, reduce your cholesterol, and hopefully your PSA level, too. However, if you do prefer a fiber bar, look for one that is generally less than 150 calories/628 kj and contains about 10 grams of mostly insoluble fiber.

Fish Oil (Omega-3 fatty acids)

Several studies have suggested that taking fish oil pills containing the two primary fish oils, EPA and DHA (500 mg–1 gram per day), may reduce the risk of sudden cardiac death and may reduce the risk of other cardiovascular events. In addition, fish oil may reduce triglycerides, which may be increased in men on some treatments for prostate cancer, and may have anti-arthritic and anti-cancer properties as well as other important benefits. Fish oil pills tend to be low in mercury. However, keep in mind that even fish oils come with a catch. They may thin your blood too much and increase your risk of internal bleeding. Please discuss with your doctor whether or not you qualify for a fish oil supplement. Individuals already on another blood-thinning medication have to be careful when combining it with fish oil pills.

Lycopene

There have been only a few studies of men taking lycopene supplements for prostate cancer prevention or with

DR. MOYAD'S FAST FAVES
Foods Rich in Lycopene
Tomatoes
Watermelon
Guava
Pink Grapefruit
Papaya
Apricots

conventional treatment, and the results thus far are inconclusive and controversial. More studies are desperately needed, but in the meantime, I am not a big supporter of lycopene dietary supplements for prostate cancer. Generally I would suggest getting more lycopene from food rather than supplements.

Multivitamins

One of the largest studies of men taking a single pill, low-dose multivitamin once a day seemed to show it prevented prostate cancer, but another study showed that men taking 2 or more multivitamin pills a day had a higher risk for advanced and fatal prostate cancer! In other words, less is more when it comes to multivitamins. It is possible that higher doses of these pills may feed prostate tumors. The real problem is that many men's multivitamins contain too high a concentration of antioxidants. Taking a children's multivitamin several times a week, not to exceed one multivitamin pill a day, makes more sense.

Read the label carefully on any multivitamin you are considering taking to see how much of key ingredients it provides. Remember that the percent daily value (% DV) or the Recommended Daily Allowance (RDA) should be the maximum (not the minimum) amount of the ingredient you need from a combination of diet and supplements. Please be most careful about folic acid and zinc in higher amounts than the DV or RDA, because they have been associated with a higher risk of aggressive prostate cancer in some of the largest human studies. Be especially careful of any multivitamin that asks you to take more than one pill a day. It is a good rule of thumb to discuss any supplement you are considering with your healthcare provider and this includes vitamins.

Probiotic Dietary Supplements

Probiotics are the so-called friendly bacteria that are advertised for immune health and promoted by some companies as being completely safe. Friendly bacteria do have a good track record for safety in foods that carry them, such as yogurt or a yogurt drink. My rule of thumb is that I do not consider any pill safe for a prostate cancer patient unless it has been tested in prostate cancer patients specifically. Probiotics in food seem fine, but we have no idea if taking these supplements after being diagnosed with cancer can help, harm, or do nothing. Also, getting millions of these bacteria may overwhelm your immune system and not stimulate it. You need a strong immune system to fight your prostate cancer, particularly because many of our best conventional medicines rely on a person having a normal immune system. While there have been some preliminary results related to bladder cancer benefits, I simply am not a supporter of probiotic supplements for patients diagnosed with or treated for prostate cancer until someone can show that they are safe and actually help.

Quercetin

This is a compound found in grapes, garlic, and other natural sources, which has some anti-inflammatory properties. We have no idea if it helps to prevent or treat prostate cancer, but it has been used with some success in treating chronic nonbacterial prostatitis. This type of pain and inflammation of the prostate is more common than previously realized. One of the most clinically tested and utilized products in the world is Q-Urol (www.Qurol.com). However, first check with your doctor to see if you even qualify for it. It is not uncommon to combine quercetin with prescription medication for chronic nonbacterial prostatitis. Quercetin is also being studied for blood pressure reduction, but it is too early to know if it has any major impact in these areas.

Saw Palmetto & Other BPH Supplements

Saw Palmetto is one of the most popular herbal products around the world used to provide some relief for the symptoms of benign prostatic hyperplasia (BPH). In a recent large clinical trial, the most commonly used dosage (320 to 960 mg per day) was very safe but worked no better than a placebo. However, a placebo works well for some men with mild BPH (no kidding).

There is no strong human research for using saw palmetto to prevent or treat prostate cancer. There is a concern that higher doses of saw palmetto may artificially reduce PSA blood levels and, in my opinion, this can happen in some men at the higher doses. Other, less popular BPH herbal products or natural remedies such as beta-sitosterol, pygeum africanum, rye pollen, and stinging nettle do not have as much research as saw palmetto and need to be tested more to see if they work better than a placebo. (I believe they do work well for some individuals.)

The biggest problem that all of these herbal products have is that the prescription medications for BPH work so well today that they are widely used. Most men who use the herbal supplement take it along with prescription medication, with their doctor's approval, of course.

Selenium

In the most recent and largest clinical trial, selenium dietary supplements did NOT work to prevent prostate cancer at a dosage of 200 mcg per day, and they may have increased the risk of type II diabetes! However, another recent

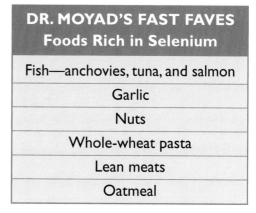

DR. MOYAD'S FAST FAVES Foods Rich in Selenium
Fish—anchovies, tuna, and salmon
Garlic
Nuts
Whole-wheat pasta
Lean meats
Oatmeal

clinical trial may have found a benefit in getting smaller amounts of selenium from healthy food sources and a vitamin and mineral combination supplement (low-dose multivitamin). Therefore, there is no reason right now to take an individual selenium supplement because it is not heart healthy and not beneficial in larger amounts. Some children's and women's multivitamins contain from 10 to 100 mcg of selenium per pill and this is more than enough. The current recommended daily allowance for men and women is only 55 mcg per day and there are plenty of healthy food sources of selenium.

Tea and Tea Supplements

Most forms of tea, including black, green, herbal, and oolong, are healthy and have few or no calories, so enjoy drinking them. However, please keep in mind that tea-based dietary supplements or pills (not the drink) have no solid proof from human studies that they do anything against prostate cancer. A large clinical trial of high-dose green tea supplements in patients with advanced cancer showed no real benefit. Patients on warfarin (a prescription blood thinner) should be careful to avoid getting large amounts of green tea because it can be a significant source of vitamin K and can reduce the efficacy of this popular blood-thinning drug.

Testosterone-Lowering Supplements

If your PSA drops significantly over a short period of time after taking a dietary supplement, talk to your doctor about getting a total testosterone and/or estrogen (estradiol) blood test. Over the last 20 years, I have witnessed several expensive dietary supplements contaminated with high concentrations of estrogen and/or estrogenlike plants that simply reduce testosterone and/or increase estrogen and thus cause a large drop in PSA over a short time. The problem with these supplements is that they not only can cost you a lot of money but they can also be life-threatening in some cases. There is such a large amount of estrogen-like material in some of these nonregulated pills that they increase breast size, cause breast pain, and increase the risk of blood clots and death. Basically, these are a costly scam or rip-off.

In the United States and around the world, there are several instances of this problem. For example, in the United States there was a dietary supplement called "PC-SPES," which cost patients thousands of dollars in some cases and caused some of the earlier mentioned side effects. It was later found through laboratory analysis to contain high amounts of estrogen-like compounds. It was removed from the market but numerous similar products have entered the marketplace, so be careful, please.

Vitamin C

Ascorbic acid or vitamin C is one of the most popular dietary supplements around the world, but researchers have not found that it helps prevent prostate cancer. There has been some interest in taking megadoses (1000s of milligrams) of this vitamin from pills or even intravenously from a doctor, but the research that this may help is weak, and it can cost you a fortune. Most of the studies of megadoses used patients with advanced or even terminal cancer. In some cases, it made patients feel better, but it had no impact on improving their survival rate. Also, the research on vitamin C to improve immune health or reduce the risk of cold or lung infection has seen the most benefit at a moderate dosage (about 500 mg per day).

Because of its acidity, vitamin C can upset your stomach. However, there are now non-acidic options of this vitamin sold as dietary supplements. Called calcium ascorbate, or buffered vitamin C, or pH neutral vitamin C, these may be a good alternative for individuals who cannot tolerate plain vitamin C. In addition, these non-acidic versions of vitamin C may be associated with a lower risk of other possible long-term side effects (compared to plain vitamin C), such as kidney stones.

Vitamin E

Most non-smokers (or ex-smokers) need only 15 to 30 mg (or IU) of natural or synthetic vitamin E to normalize their blood levels. You can get this amount from a children's multivitamin and/or from healthy foods, particularly nuts, seeds, and plant-based cooking oils.

Zinc & Other Eye-Health Supplements

Zinc has been promoted as an eye-healthy, immune-healthy, and prostate-healthy dietary supplement. However, zinc supplements in high dosages, 80 to 100 mg/day or more, should be avoided by most men and women, in my opinion. Recent human research has linked higher doses of zinc from dietary supplements to abnormal immune changes, a potential reduction in the impact of bone-building drugs, abnormal changes in the cholesterol blood tests, increased risk of urinary tract infections, kidney stones, prostate enlargement, and an increased risk of aggressive prostate cancer. Some government health organizations (Canada, for example) no longer allow the sale of high-dose zinc in a single pill based on this new research.

Normally, only 0.5 mg of zinc is lost from the body every day, and this is easily replaced by dietary sources. Keep in mind that most good cheap multivitamins contain about 10–20 mg of zinc, which is more than enough for most men with just one exception. Men taking zinc supplements for eye health, or more specifically the dry form of age-related macular degeneration (AMD), should not take more than 80 mg of zinc per day from these supplements. This was the dosage, along with other antioxidants (500 mg vitamin C, 400 IU vitamin E, 15 mg beta-carotene, and 2 mg cupric oxide), that may have reduced the risk of vision loss in individuals with moderate to severe forms of AMD. So, if there is an issue of preserving your sight because of your AMD, your cancer and eye doctors should both agree first and foremost that you need zinc in higher doses, along with other antioxidants, before you take these eye-health supplements.

A Final Note on Supplements

When I speak with patients, my general advice is that 2 to 3 weeks before any surgical or radiation procedure patients should discontinue the use of almost all dietary supplements. Preliminary evidence has demonstrated that some supplements may thin your blood during surgery, may interact with the anesthetic used in surgery, or may reduce the impact of radiation or other conventional treatments. Therefore, in order to be safe rather than sorry, it is best to focus on healthy lifestyle and dietary changes during this time. When you have recovered from surgery or have completed radiation or other conventional treatments, then you and your doctor should discuss when it is okay to restart the use of certain dietary supplements. This general rule should also apply to chemotherapy or other treatments.

Please keep in mind that most other dietary supplements are not needed at this time. Always have a discussion with your doctor before conventional prostate cancer treatment begins about which supplements are and are not appropriate during this time. For example, some doctors advise vitamin D supplementation with some chemotherapy drugs and others do not. Again, as always, the ultimate decision about which dietary supplements to discontinue or maintain during conventional prostate cancer treatment should be between you and your doctor.

Prescription Drugs

In addition to the supplements just discussed, a few general prescription drugs are worth noting here.

Cholesterol-, Blood Pressure-, and Blood Sugar-Lowering Medications

The amazing thing about cholesterol-lowering medications (statins) is that they not only seem to reduce the risk of cardiovascular disease, but they recently have been associated with better prostate health and may improve your prognosis during and after treatment for prostate cancer. Statins may also increase vitamin D blood levels. The same findings have been suggested for blood pressure and blood sugar-reducing (diabetes) medications. This requires further study. If you cannot get your cholesterol, blood pressure, or blood sugar levels down to normal levels with healthy lifestyle changes, then do not be shy about asking your doctor about some of these medications that may help.

Metformin, a generic blood sugar control drug used to treat type 2 diabetes, has been shown to prevent diabetes and help with weight loss in some prostate cancer patients. It is also being studied as an anti-cancer agent and preliminary evidence suggests it may prevent or slow the growth of prostate tumors.

There is a dietary supplement known as "red yeast rice extract" that has helped reduce cholesterol in the small number of individuals who are not able to take any of the statin medications. However, this dietary supplement contains one of the active ingredients found in an actual statin, so patients on this supplement should be monitored (liver and muscle enzyme studies) as if they are on a statin. I generally recommend statins first as opposed to this supplement because they have the clinical research, are covered by insurance, are getting cheaper, and have a great safety record.

Dutasteride, Finasteride (5-alpha-reductase inhibitors), and Other BPH Prescription Medications (alpha-blockers)

New research is emerging to suggest dutasteride and finasteride, also known as the 5-alpha-reductase inhibitors, may not only reduce your risk of prostate cancer but may help to partially treat the disease along with conventional treatment. These drugs are used in some men with non-cancerous enlargement of the prostate or benign prostatic hyperplasia (BPH) because they actually shrink the prostate over time and work especially well in men with large prostates. Dutasteride and finasteride can reduce a man's PSA level by up to 50 percent over six months. However, whether or not these pills can help treat prostate cancer as well as they can prevent prostate cancer is still controversial. They may prevent non-aggressive prostate cancers and even treat some of them when a man is on active surveillance. However, they increase the risk of sexual dysfunction and, in rare circumstances; they may increase the risk of more aggressive prostate cancer. You should talk to your doctor about the latest research on these and other BPH medications because numerous large clinical trials are going on now in the prevention and treatment setting. In addition to treating BPH, finasteride is used at a lower dosage in several countries to prevent hair loss or premature balding. Even at the lower dosage, it can reduce a man's PSA level.

Another class of BPH medications, alpha-blockers, relaxes the prostate in men with BPH and may have some cancer-preventive effects. These drugs generally work faster to improve urinary problems in men with BPH, but their anti-cancer effects are not as well established and they do not generally cause a large reduction in PSA. Some men with severe BPH take both types of drugs to help relieve their symptoms, but the vast majority of men with BPH take one or the other drug.

Weight-Loss Prescription Drugs

For the first time in almost 15 years, there will be new prescription weight-loss drugs available for men and women in the United States. If weight is a concern, please discuss the new options with your doctor.

The following table provides a quick overview of many supplements and prescription medications that patients regularly ask about.

Supplement or Medication	Comments
Aspirin	Low-dose baby aspirin only makes sense for those with a higher risk of heart disease.
Beta-Sitosterol, Pygeum Africanum, or Saw Palmetto	All possible options for non-cancerous enlargement of the prostate (BPH) with or without prescription medications. Not known if they fight cancer or not.
B-Complex Vitamin Supplement	Avoid these because they may encourage tumor growth in some men.
Calcium	If any concern exists about bone health and you cannot get enough from foods and beverages, take calcium supplements, but those with a history of calcium stones need to take calcium citrate.
Coenzyme Q10 (CoQ10)	May provide a slight benefit in reducing the side effects of cholesterol-lowering drugs, otherwise there is no need to take an individual CoQ10 supplement.

Supplement or Medication	Comments
Fish Oil	One of the best supplements for any man with prostate cancer to reduce triglycerides, arthritis pain, and prevent weight gain. It is eye and heart healthy. If you cannot swallow the large pill, use a flavored liquid form.
Flaxseed or Soy Dietary Supplements (plant estrogen supplement)	Most of the research is with the food sources (powder or protein powder), so stay away from the dietary supplement options.
Ginger	One of the best dietary supplements to take (500 to 1000 mg per day) to reduce nausea during and after chemotherapy.
Glucosamine, Pycnogenol, or SAM-e Dietary Supplements	Taken for osteoarthritis, has a very good safety record. Now available in liquid options, but has no evidence in prostate cancer treatment.
Green Tea Supplements	Skip the supplements (has no research) and simply drink green tea. It has zero calories, a moderate amount of healthy caffeine, an anti-stress compound (L-theanine), and other healthy nutrients. Can be consumed cold or hot.

Supplement or Medication	Comments
Korean Red Ginseng (Panax Ginseng), MACA, or L-arginine aspartate & pycnogenol	These options have very good preliminary data to show they improve sexual health (erectile function/libido) in men and Panax ginseng even has data to support it potentially helps women, but there are serious quality-control issues with these products so try and find a reputable company.
Lutein and Zeaxanthin	These eye health supplements may help those with macular degeneration (one of the leading causes of vision loss) but have no evidence in prostate cancer.
Metformin	Generic drug shown to prevent diabetes and help with weight loss in prostate cancer patients and may have anti-cancer benefit.
Multivitamin	Take one children's multivitamin per day day maximum if you want a multivitamin.
Niacin (vitamin B3)	One of the only B-vitamins that some individuals need to take in larger amounts in an over the counter or prescription form to increase HDL and lower triglycerides. Stay away from "no flush" niacin and just use "immediate-release" or prescription extended release niacin,

Supplement or Medication	Comments
Niacin (vitamin B3) con't	if needed at all.
Panax quinquefolius (also known American Ginseng)	This dietary supplement (1000 to 2000 mg per as day) has helped some patients reduce their fatigue and improve energy levels during chemotherapy or other cancer treatments. Should not be taken during localized prostate cancer treatment because it may have blood- thinning or blood glucose-lowering effects.
Probiotics (healthy bacteria) supplements	Should be avoided by most cancer patients because of the lack of research Getting lots of fiber already gives you healthy bacteria. The only exception to my avoidance rule is with bladder cancer or bladder health. There, clinical trials find that a type of healthy bacteria from yogurt may provide a treatment benefit.
Resveratrol	This so-called anti-aging compound is sold as a supplement, but red wine is actually the best source of this compound.
Selenium	Stay away from individual supplements. Enough is provided by a children's multivitamin.

Supplement or Medication	Comments
Statin (cholesterol-lowering prescription drug)	Should be a consideration for anyone anyone with prostate cancer who is not able to lower cholesterol andhs-CRP blood test enough using diet and exercise alone. Statins come with short- and long-term side effects so be careful to always go with the lowest effective dosage (if needed).
Vitamin C	Get it from a multivitamin. Or, higher amounts (500 to 1000 mg per day) for immune health (colds) are safe, but try to take a non-acidic form if you are concerned about side effects.
Vitamin D	Take about 800 to 1000 IU (25 mcg) of vitamin D3 (also known as "cholecalciferol") every day on average. You can get a vitamin D blood test (25-OH vitamin D) to see how much vitamin D you need.
Vitamin E	Do not take this supplement by itself in any form. Just get your vitamin E from food or a children's multivitamin.

Supplement or Medication	Comments
Whey Protein or Other Protein Powder (egg white, casein, soy, brown rice, pea, hemp, etc.)	Can be taken as a powdered drink supplement (never as a pill) for any man needing more high-quality protein for health, weight loss, and to support muscle health.
Zinc	There is no need to take an individual zinc supplement (prostate unhealthy), just get it in your children's multivitamin.

CHECK IT OUT! To print a copy of the supplement chart to discuss with your physician, visit www.sprypubprostate.com.

Other Considerations for a Healthy Lifestyle

Sleep

In a recent study, researchers found that when it comes to overall impact on quality of life, sleep disruption during cancer treatment is highly significant. Researchers noted many causes of sleep disturbance, from surgical site tenderness to hot flashes caused by treatments and anxiety about treatment prognosis, and they also found that patients felt that restful sleep was important to their treatment outcome. Of course, everyone experiences sleep disturbances at times, but it is important to discuss any regular sleep interruptions with your doctor. There are behavioral, psychological, over-the-counter, and even prescription medications available to help provide more restful sleep.

Sexuality

When a man faces a prostate cancer diagnosis, concerns over sexuality often worry both him and his partner. While questions may abound, sexuality is an area where you may not be quite as comfortable asking your healthcare worker for answers. It doesn't hurt to start your research online because you can read about other prostate cancer patient's experiences. Then, follow up with some specific questions for your doctor. He or she can offer many options to help with any physical or emotional challenges. While the topic is too broad for us to cover in a book of this size, we will discuss erectile dysfunction specifically in the side effects chapter. With some patience and persistence, you and your partner will work together through your recovery following any treatment.

Did you know?

Heart Healthy = Erection Healthy. Exercise, blood pressure, cholesterol lowering, weight loss ... all can help to improve blood flow to the penis.

Vaccines

On a topic often ignored by adults—talk to your doctor

about updating your vaccines. It could improve both the quality and quantity of your life. The flu, pneumococcal, and shingles vaccines are commonly missed in men with prostate cancer (or men in general). Here is a list of some of the vaccines you can review with your primary care doctor to see if you are up to date:

- Flu shot (influenza vaccine): annually in the early fall season
- Hepatitis A and/or B: if in a risk group
- Measles-mumps-rubella vaccine: once, if born after 1956 and not immune
- Pneumococcal vaccine: at age 65 or sooner if risk factors are present
- Shingles vaccine: if age 60 years or older (or earlier if in a high-risk group) and you never had shingles, some individuals may qualify even if they have had shingles
- Tetanus-diphtheria (Td) booster: every 10 years
- Varicella (Chicken Pox) vaccine: if not immune

Other Screening Tests

It may seem strange to consider screening tests for other illnesses here, but they can be important to your overall wellness. Colon cancer is the third most common cause of cancer death in men (after lung and prostate cancer). And, screening for colon cancer with a colonoscopy has the potential to cure you during the actual screening procedure. Doctors can remove colon polyps during the procedure in some cases, and this can help to reduce your risk of developing colon cancer. Imagine if all of the cancer screening tests allowed you to be potentially cured while the doctor was screening you for the disease. Generally, men and women age 50 and older qualify for colon cancer screening. If there is a family history of the disease, some doctors like to start screening at the age of 40, and I could not agree more with this. There are several different methods used for colon cancer screening, from testing for blood in the stool, to laboratory testing, to imaging, to sigmoidoscopy and colonoscopy. Ask your doctor about the screening test that is right for you, but for most individuals I recommend a colonoscopy.

At least in some countries, a new screening test approved for men aged 65–75 years who ever smoked is abdominal aortic aneurysm (AAA) screening. It is done one time with an ultrasound, a device that is safe and gives off no radiation. Talk to your doctor to see if you qualify.

Other important screening tests—hearing, sight, skin cancer, and others—need to be handled on an individual basis. There are so many screening tests today that deciding which ones are important for an individual should be based on discussions with a trusted doctor. High priority screenings will focus on what has the greatest chance of reducing one's quality and quantity of life.

Mental Wellness

It seems fitting to end our discussion on promotion overall wellness by considering mental wellness. There is no disputing that a diagnosis of cancer and the possibility of undergoing cancer treatment add stress to lives that already have a full set of regular challenges. Anxiety and depression are common among patients during and following cancer treatment. Patients and caregivers need to look out for signs of stress and be ready to ask for or offer help. There are many resources available—from support groups, to other patients, to mental health professionals—and one is sure to fit with the patient's needs. Be sure to discuss any concerns with your healthcare professional.

From Diagnosis to Grading and Staging

In this section, we'll provide a quick guide to be used with your doctor to discuss anything from the anatomy of the prostate gland to biopsy to grading (aggressiveness of your cancer) and staging (location of your cancer). It is an overview designed to help you better understand your prostate cancer, how it is acting, and where it may be located. Please use this material with your physician.

Anatomy

Your prostate sits deep in the pelvic area of the body. It consists of 3 zones: the peripheral zone or PZ (65–70 percent of the total area of the prostate), the central zone or CZ (20–25 percent of the total area of the prostate), and the transition zone or TZ (5–10 percent of the total area of the prostate). Most prostate cancers begin growing in the PZ, and this is the area or zone that can be felt by

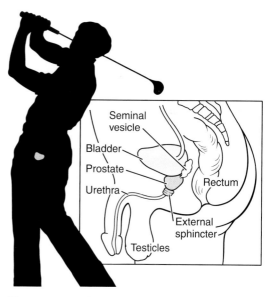

The prostate sits deep within the pelvic area of the body.

the doctor during the digital rectal exam (DRE). The DRE only takes seconds. Prostate cancer less frequently grows in the CZ and TZ. The TZ surrounds the urethra, the part of the body that carries urine from the bladder to the penis. The

TZ is where benign prostatic hyperplasia (BPH) or non-cancerous enlargement of the prostate occurs. BPH is common and can cause urinary problems. Please discuss with your healthcare professional the specifics of prostate anatomy.

Blood and Urine Tests

There are several versions of the Prostate Specific Antigen (PSA) blood test and a new urine test that you and your doctor may want to discuss. The lower the PSA value over time the better, and this includes before and after diagnosis and treatment. Keep in mind that every test, including the PSA, comes with a catch and you should ask your doctor about the test, the accuracy of the test, and specific risks whenever he or she recommends having a test done.

PSA (Prostate Specific Antigen)

This blood test used to be considered normal when your PSA level was below 4 ng/ml, but newer research has revealed that a man can have cancer at any PSA level. Although it is more likely that cancer is involved with a higher PSA value, it should be kept in mind that BPH and even an infection of the prostate can raise the PSA level significantly. Following a sudden large increase in PSA over a short time, some doctors will first give the patient a course of antibiotics that last on average for 4 weeks to see if the PSA comes down quickly, indicating that an infection existed. If antibiotics are not the answer, the doctor begins to look for cancer or other possible reasons for the increase in the PSA.

Many doctors are now relying on the way PSA changes over time (also known as "PSA kinetics") in combination with age, family history, race, weight, DRE, and, at times, imaging tests to determine if a man should have a biopsy or if there is a possibility that cancer is in the prostate. The value of PSA is not only checked before diagnosis, but especially after diagnosis and treatment.

Recently, there has been controversy over when (or if) a man should have a routine PSA test done. It can be confusing, so men should discuss the pros and cons of the test with their physicians to make a decision based on the man's individual situation.

PSA Density (PSAD = PSA/size of the prostate)

If you have had your PSA measured and have also received a transrectal ultrasound (TRUS) around the same time, this can help to determine your PSAD. TRUS, along with a DRE, is a good way to determine the size of the prostate and, when the PSA level is divided by the size or volume of the prostate, this equals PSAD. Some studies indicate that there is a greater chance of prostate cancer with a higher PSAD.

PSA Doubling Time

PSA doubling time is now viewed as important because it is the time it takes for your PSA value to double from your first PSA test. It can provide some valuable information before and after diagnosis or treatment. It can be calculated with just a few PSA tests over time, and you do not need to wait for your actual PSA to double in order to predict or calculate with your doctor how quickly it will double. The faster a PSA doubles, the more likely that your cancer is on the move.

PSA Velocity (PSAV)

This measurement is relevant because it is the determination of how quickly the PSA is rising over a certain period of time. At least 2 to 3 individual PSA tests are needed over 6 months to a year to calculate this value. A higher PSAV over a period of time is more of an indication of cancer as compared to a low PSAV. For example, if your PSA goes from 1 to 3 ng/ml in one year (PSAV = 2), this is more of a concern compared to one that goes from 1 to 1.5 ng/ml (PSAV = 0.5). It can also provide valuable information about your cancer before and after treatment.

Free-to-Total PSA Blood Test

This test or a version of it can help the doctor decide if you need a biopsy when the situation is not quite clear. The greater the percentage of free PSA in the blood compared to PSA that is bound to something else, the greater the chance that you are "free" of cancer. So, a man with a free PSA of 35% is less likely to have cancer as compared to one who has a free PSA of 10%. This test this should only be used when the decision to biopsy or not is unclear.

ProsVue Test

This FDA-approved blood test can be used after having surgery to remove the prostate. The test helps to predict the risk of cancer coming back after this surgical procedure which is why it is also known as a "post-radical prostatectomy prognostic test." ProsVue is an immunoassay to quantify very low levels of PSA. The assay can detect levels in picograms (a trillionth) per mL in men after radical prostatectomy to help identify men at a low risk of clinical recurrence. It has a limit of quantification of 0.000065 ng/mL (0.65 pg/mL) or 10 times below the detection limit of most tests. This test attempts to assist in the prediction, along with other clinical information, of who will or will not have a recurrence of their prostate cancer within 8 years of their surgery. It may be most helpful for men with high risk pathology after surgery to help them decide for example if they want radiation treatment at some point.

Testosterone Blood Test

Testosterone blood testing (usually more accurate if the blood draw is done in the morning) needs to be requested more by patients and some physicians. It is easy to get fixated on PSA blood testing, but some of the most common treatments for prostate cancer (androgen deprivation therapy) rely on having a castration or low level of testosterone. If testosterone impacts PSA, weight loss, libido, energy levels, and even possibly treatments...why aren't we asking about this test more often?

Urine Tests (PROGENSA® PCA3 Test and Others)

The new PROSENSA PCA3 test helps some clinicians

determine the need for a repeat biopsy after an initial negative biopsy, but it is not suggested for use if the previous biopsy had atypical small acinar proliferation (ASAP), a type of pre-cancerous lesion. ASAP is associated with a 40 to 50 percent chance of having cancer diagnosed on a subsequent biopsy and repeat biopsies are recommended if ASAP is identified.

In general, these urine tests are done in the office and may require some prostatic massage by the doctor to get a sample. The tests are usually offered for men whose PSA and other tests have not provided a clear enough idea of whether or not a biopsy is needed or if cancer might be present. The higher the score on the urine tests, the higher the chance that you have cancer.

Imaging Tests Used in Prostate Cancer

A variety of imaging tests are used to give physicians a re-liable analysis of the location and possible spread of your can-cer. Many of these tests are used to provide a baseline when compared to the same test at a later date. For example, com-paring a recent bone scan to a bone scan from months or years ago can help determine if bone metastasis or further spread of the cancer has occurred. These tests may lead to further tests or treatments, such as a biopsy, the removal of a lymph node, or the treatment of an area of the body to elim-inate tumor cells. Most of these imaging procedures are pain-less, with the possible exception of a needle stick to inject dye to improve readability of results.

Bone Scan

A bone scan, also called a "radionuclide bone scan" or "bone scintigraphy," is the gold standard test for determining if a patient has prostate cancer that has spread to any of the bones. The test exposes the patient to radiation and may not be able to pick up very tiny bone metastasis. It can appear falsely positive for cancer if the patient has arthritis, degenerative bone disease, infection, or fracture.

Computed Tomography (CT scan)

A CT scan can find cancer in the regional and non-regional lymph nodes, especially when the nodes become large in size because the test detects this size change. It is a good complementary test to investigate a suspicious region found on bone scan or plain x-ray. The test exposes the patient to radiation and until the lymph node becomes larger in size it cannot detect a possible cancer in that location.

Intravenous Pyelogram (IVP)

An IVP is used to provide an image of the kidneys, ureters, and bladder. The test exposes the patient to radiation. It is rarely used any more because newer devices are preferred.

Magnetic Resonance Imaging (MRI)

An MRI does not involve exposure to radiation. It may be able to find cancer in and around the prostate, such as the seminal vesicles or regional lymph nodes. MRI can even find tumors in the spine, especially some high-grade tumors. MRI is not good at detecting cancer in the lymph nodes unless a special iron oxide dye is used. It is not as useful as bone scan for finding cancer in bony areas. Because the test utilizes a strong magnet, it cannot be used on individuals with metal in their bodies, such as from past medical procedures.

PET/CT Scan

This technology is rapidly developing. It may be able to pick up cancer in the organs, bone, or non-regional and regional lymph node metastasis very early when the nodes are still not large enough to be picked up by CT scan or MRI. It can sometimes detect cancer when a bone scan did not find cancer in the bones because it relies on a tracer compound to find even tiny tumors. The patient is exposed to radiation. Finding the right tracer marker (carbon-11, choline, glucose, NaF) to be used with the test is challenging because the technology is developing so quickly. In some cases, patients have problems with insurance coverage for this test.

ProstaScint Scan

The ProstaScint scan can suggest whether or not cancer has returned after localized treatment for prostate cancer, especially in the areas around the prostate. This test is of little value for a man with hormone refractory prostate cancer. Also, the accuracy of this test has been questioned.

Transrectal Ultrasonography (TRUS)

A TRUS involves no radiation exposure. It is the gold

standard device to obtain prostate tissue biopsy samples. The TRUS is not a good test by itself for detecting a tumor in or near the prostate.

X-ray

In traditional x-ray procedures, the patient receives a low amount of radiation exposure. The tests can be done quickly. X-rays only show something when it is more obvious and takes up a lot of space, such as an infection, fracture, or cancer in the lungs or the ribs. They are not as good at finding small-to-moderate amounts of cancer or bone loss.

The Prostate Biopsy

It is impossible for most individuals to be diagnosed with prostate cancer without a sample of prostate tissue or a biopsy. During the biopsy, the doctor will take numerous samples (also called "cores") from different areas of the prostate. The number of samples taken depends on your situation and your doctor. The standard number used to be 6, but better detection has been achieved by in-

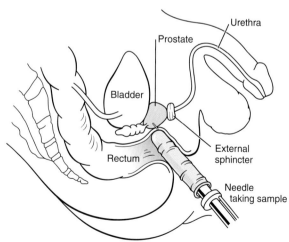

Using a needle, a biopsy takes samples of prostate tissue that will then be reviewed by a pathologist.

creasing the number of samples in some cases to 12 or more.

Regardless of the number of samples, a pathologist reads them and decides whether each and every sample taken has normal cells, cancerous cells, and/or something that is not cancerous but is also not quite normal in appearance. Since a biopsy can reveal more than just cancer present, I recommend that every man keep a copy of his biopsy report. An example of a 6-core and 12-core biopsy follows. Notice how the report not only shows the location of the sample that has cancer, but it also quantifies the percentage of the sample taken that actually had cancerous cells in it. The amount of cancer in each sample is important; the more cancer, the more the concern. Also keep in mind that the word impression is the medical terminology that means the "bottom line" or the "cut to the chase" part of this or most other reports from the doctor.

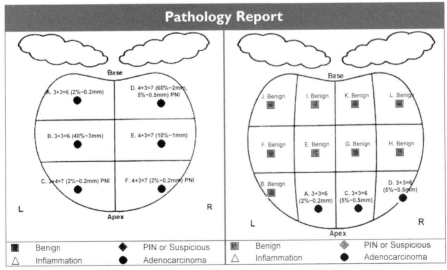

Examples of a 6-core and 12-core biopsy.

Other important information from the biopsy can include the words: "high-grade prostatic intraepithelial neoplasia (HGPIN)" or "atypical small acinar proliferation (ASAP)." These terms do not represent cancer when they are found in a biopsy sample report. Instead, they represent a gray area or "not quite cancer but not quite normal either." High-grade PIN and/or ASAP are considered pre-cancerous markers and can frequently coexist with cancer or just increase the chance that cancer will be found on a future biopsy. The greater the number of biopsy samples that contain one or both of these markers, the greater the chance of being diagnosed with cancer in the future. The doctor will often recommend a repeat biopsy in 6 to 12 months if a man has one or both of these markers. I tell patients to go over their pathology report carefully with their doctor even if the doctor says there is no cancer. It is important to know if any of the samples contained HGPIN, ASAP, or another marker that lets you know if you should be followed more closely by your doctor.

Sometimes a physician will recommend doing a "Saturation Biopsy." It is more extensive as compared to a regular biopsy and involves taking as many as 30, 40, 50, or even more samples. The patient is given anesthesia and is asleep for the procedure. This biopsy is used to get a more complete picture if results are unclear from a single biopsy or series of biopsies. There are extra risks as well as benefits so talk to your physician about the process he or she recommends for you.

Few things in prostate cancer need an independent second opinion more than a biopsy reading if there are any concerns on your or your doctor's part. Since the Gleason score is based on interpretation of the biopsy and it will be used as an indicator for what (if any) treatment you will receive in the future, it is always better to resolve any doubts that may exist at this point. For example, men who qualify for active surveillance because of their low Gleason score and small amount of tumor in the prostate may feel more comfortable with the surveillance choice if they know that a second independent pathologist agrees with the biopsy results.

If you have been diagnosed with cancer, the pathologist looking at your slides will attempt to determine how aggressive your cancer is (called "grading") and if your cancer is contained within the prostate or has spread beyond the prostate (called "staging"). Although there are always exceptions, in general, it is important to wait at least 4 to 6 weeks after a positive biopsy (one that shows cancer) to then have surgery, radiation, or another treatment because the prostate needs time to heal to reduce your potential side effects from the treatment you choose.

It is not unusual many months or years after prostate cancer radiation treatment to receive another biopsy if the doctor questions if the cancer may have returned, perhaps as suggested by a rapidly rising PSA. I agree with this choice because it gives you a better idea if cancer has indeed returned in the area that was around or near the originally radiated area.

Gleason Scores

The Gleason system is based on how effectively the cells

of any particular cancer are able to structure themselves into glands resembling those of the normal prostate. The ability of a tumor to mimic normal gland architecture is called its differentiation, and experience has shown that a tumor whose structure is nearly normal (well differentiated) will probably behave relatively close to normal—that is, not very aggressive. To determine a Gleason grade, a pathologist looks at each cancerous tissue sample and assigns it two numbers from 1 (least aggressive) to 5 (most aggressive). Two numbers are given because prostate tumors from a single individual will generally show some variation. In other words, some of the tumor might look aggressive, while some of it may not.

The first number of the Gleason score is the most common or primary predominant type of cancer in the sample and the second number is the second most common tumor type seen on the sample. For example, a 4 + 3 = 7 means a "moderately poorly differentiated" cancer as you can see in the table on page 92, but it also means that there existed more of a 4 primary pattern in the sample compared to a 3 secondary pattern. In general, the lower your total Gleason score, the less aggressive the cancer, and the higher the Gleason score the more aggressive the cancer. This also may be true of the individual numbers that make up the total score. A 4 + 3 is slightly more aggressive as compared to a 3 + 4, even though both add up to 7, because the primary or majority predominant tumor type is 4 (more aggressive) in the first case and 3 (less aggressive) in the second case. In addition, it is important that you know that it is very rare today to be diagnosed with a total Gleason score of 2 to 4, or even 5. In fact, the average or common type of prostate cancer diagnosed currently is a total Gleason score of 6 or 7. Why? Many pathologists believe that Gleason scores of 2–5 are not completely or actually cancer in some cases but have a lot of normal features. Therefore, Gleason scores of 6 and 7 now represent the majority of the prostate tumors diagnosed, and Gleason scores of 8 to 10 remain as the group of tumors that are generally more aggressive.

A summary of the potential Gleason scores that could appear on your pathology report follows in the table. Keep in mind that every single prostate biopsy sample with cancer will be assigned its own Gleason score, but please discuss what your overall Gleason score means with your doctor.

Possible Gleason Scores	
Gleason Scores	**What Does That Tell Us?**
1+1, 2+1, 1+2, 1+3 2+1, 2+2 3+1	2−4 = Well differentiated cancer or not aggressive
1+4, 1+5 2+3, 2+4 3+2, 3+3 4+1, 4+2 5+1	5−6 = Moderately differentiated cancer or moderately aggressive
2+5 3+4 4+3 5+2	7 = Moderately poorly differentiated or aggressive
3+5 4+4, 4+5 5+3, 5+4, 5+5	8−10 = Poorly differentiated cancer or very aggressive

TNM and ABCD Clinical Staging Systems

These staging systems are used to quantify the progression of prostate cancers. If you compare the staging system with the illustrations you will get an idea of what the letters are indicating. Please discuss with your doctor if your cancer has spread and where it would be ranked on this system. Keep in mind that numerous tests and not just the pathology report can be used to determine the specific location of your cancer.

In considering prostate cancer that has spread to lymph nodes, doctors are looking at nodes in 3 regions of the body. The following illustrations will give you an idea of the nodes involved in each area and the possible progression.

Clinical Staging Systems for Localized Prostate Cancer		
TNM	**ABCD**	**What do the results mean?**
TX	—	The cancer cannot be staged at this time.
T0	—	There is no evidence of a cancer.
T1	A	A cancer that cannot be felt with a DRE or picked up by an imaging machine (X-ray, CT scan, MRI, etc.) or is found by PSA or another procedure, such as a TURP for BPH. This is "localized or confined prostate cancer."
T1a	A1	A cancer that is found during a procedure such as a TURP (not found by biopsy). The cancer takes up less than 5 percent of prostate tissue removed in the procedure.
T1b	A2	A cancer that is found during a procedure such as a TURP. The cancer takes up more than 5 percent of the prostate tissue removed in the procedure.
T1c	B0	A cancer that cannot be felt with a DRE but it is detected by biopsy in one or both sides of the prostate, because of an initial high PSA level.
T2	B1 or B2	The cancer is only confined or within the prostate, and/or it has invaded the apex of the prostate (where the urethra leaves the prostate), or it has gone into but not beyond the prostate capsule. This is still called a "localized or confined prostate cancer."

T1a

Bladder

Rectum

Prostate

Exam Finger

T1b

T1c

PSA   PSA

PSA

Clinical Staging Systems for Advanced Prostate Cancer			
T2a	B1	A cancer that occupies only one side (lobe) of the prostate.	T2a
T2b	B2	A cancer that occupies both sides (lobes) of the prostate.	
TNM	ABCD	What do the results mean?	
T3	C1-C2	The cancer goes through the prostate capsule. This is also called "locally advanced prostate disease."	T2b
T3a	C1	A cancer on one or both sides of the prostate that is now growing on the outside and going beyond the prostate. This is also called "unilateral (one side) or bilateral (both sides) extracapsular extension."	T3a
T3b	C2	A cancer that has invaded one or both seminal vesicles.	
T4	C2	A cancer that has spread to or invaded other nearby structures other than the seminal vesicle(s), such as the: bladder neck, external sphincter, rectum, nearby muscles (also called "levator muscles") and/or the pelvic wall. This is also called a "locally or regionally advanced prostate cancer."	T3b

Clinical Staging Systems for Advanced Prostate Cancer

NX	—	The lymph nodes cannot be staged at this time.
N0	—	No lymph nodes near the prostate have cancer (or metastasis). These are also called "regional lymph nodes."
N1	D1	Cancer in a regional node or nodes near the prostate. This is also called a "regionally advanced prostate cancer."
MX	—	Metastasis or cancer spread far beyond the prostate (also called "distant metastasis") cannot be staged at this time.
M0	—	There is no metastasis or cancer spread far beyond the prostate (also called "no distant metastasis").
M1	D2	Cancer has metastasized or spread far beyond the prostate (also called "distant metastasis"). This is also called "advanced prostate cancer."
M1a	D2	Cancer has metastasized or spread to a node or nodes far beyond the prostate (also called "nonregional lymph node or nodes").
M1b	D2	Cancer has metastasized or spread to the bone(s).
M1c	D2	Cancer has metastasized or spread to another site or sites in the body far beyond the prostate (such as liver, lungs, and bones). This is the most advanced category or stage of prostate cancer.

Pelvic Nodes

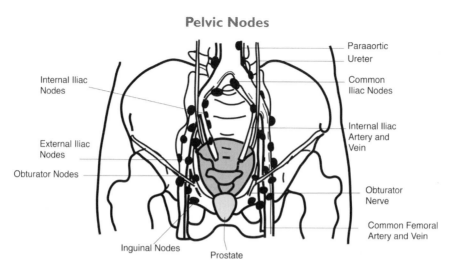

Paraaortic
Ureter
Internal Iliac Nodes
Common Iliac Nodes
Internal Iliac Artery and Vein
External Iliac Nodes
Obturator Nodes
Obturator Nerve
Common Femoral Artery and Vein
Inguinal Nodes
Prostate

The pelvic lymph nodes are the first set of nodes in the human body where prostate cancer usually goes after growing beyond the prostate area.

Abdominal Nodes

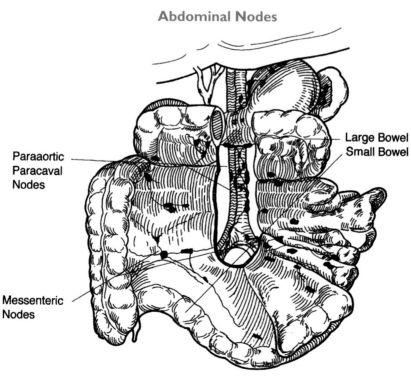

Paraaortic Paracaval Nodes
Large Bowel
Small Bowel
Messenteric Nodes

The abdominal pelvic lymph nodes are the second set of nodes where cancer may typically spread.

Peri Hilar/Supraclavicular Nodes

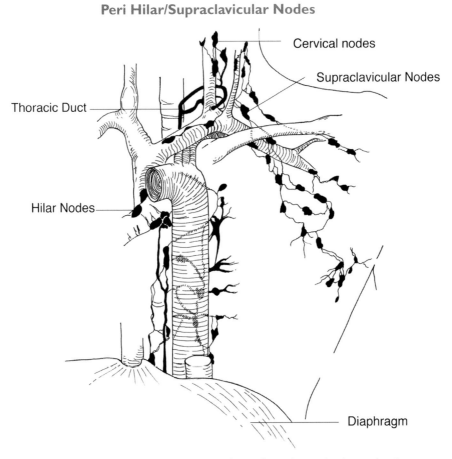

The Peri Hilar/Supraclavicular lymph nodes, located generally speaking in the chest and neck area, are usually the third set of nodes where prostate cancer spreads.

A Final Note

After reviewing test results and grading and staging your cancer, a treatment plan will be developed. Your doctor will work with you to consider all the information about your cancer and discuss what she or he feels is the best option for your individual situation. While it may be an unsettling and, at times, confusing conversation, it is important to ask any questions you may have and take time to consider the choices. If you are unsure of what course you should take, you may want to get an independent second opinion to be sure that you are comfortable with your treatment plan. In the next section of the book, we'll provide an overview of current treatment options.

Section Three
Treatment Options

Once the grade and stage of your prostate cancer are determined, the doctor might summarize your prostate cancer risk category or group as being low, intermediate, or high, which helps to determine the risk of cancer spreading or even returning at some point in the future after treatment. The reason your cancer may be placed in one of these three categories is that it helps you and your doctor decide how aggressive you want to be with your treatment. For example, high-risk patients may receive multiple treatments such as surgery or radiation with androgen deprivation treatment (ADT). Lower risk patients might adopt a more conservative treatment such as active surveillance.

Risk Category/Group	PSA (ng/ml)	Gleason Score	Stage (Location)
Low (all of the following features)	Less than 10	2–6	Tumor occupies a small area or just one side of the prostate.
Intermediate (one or more of the following features)	10–20	7	Tumor occupies a large area of one side of the prostate.
High or more of the following features)	Greater than 20	8–10	Tumor involves one or both sides of the prostate.

One of the most common questions I'm asked when speaking with patients is which type of surgery, radiation treatment, or any other treatment is best when compared to another. I often tell patients that "treatment fits personality." Since the long-term results are fairly similar between the types of surgery and/or radiation, a man impacted by prostate cancer should choose which treatment best fits him after an extensive investigation of each option and its benefits and possible drawbacks. For example, some patients like the ease of radiation therapy, but others do not like the thought that if cancer should return after radiation that most men cannot have surgery to remove the prostate. Some patients like the fact that surgery removes the whole prostate and the entire tumor, but others do not like the fact that there may be some immediate side effects and recovery time needed. You should spend some time collecting information on each treatment and then have a discussion with your doctor to develop a treatment plan that best fits your personality and situation.

Surgery

Figures A to C show where incisions are made and what steps are involved in a radical prostatectomy in both the open or traditional surgery and in a laparoscopic or robotic surgery. Figure D shows the reconstruction process following the prostatectomy. The average total time for a radical prostatectomy is 2–3 hours.

Incision types

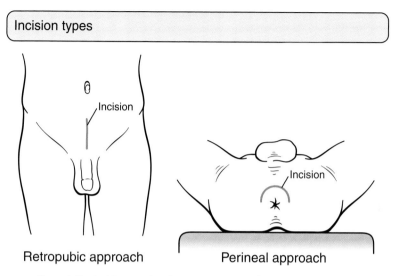

Incision

Incision

Retropubic approach   Perineal approach

Figure A. The incisions used in the two open types of radical prostatectomy.

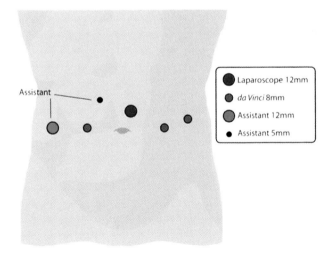

Assistant

● Laparoscope 12mm
● *da Vinci* 8mm
● Assistant 12mm
● Assistant 5mm

Figure B. The small incisions used in robotic surgery.

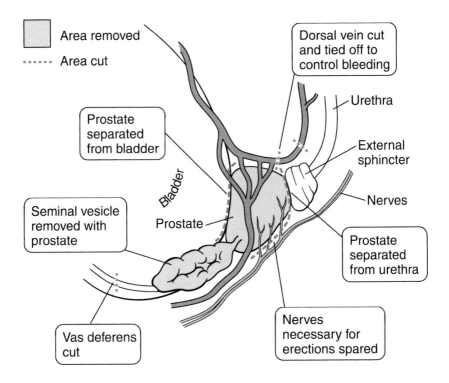

- Area removed
- Area cut

Dorsal vein cut and tied off to control bleeding

Urethra

Prostate separated from bladder

External sphincter

Bladder

Nerves

Seminal vesicle removed with prostate

Prostate

Prostate separated from urethra

Vas deferens cut

Nerves necessary for erections spared

Figure C. The prostatectomy procedure.

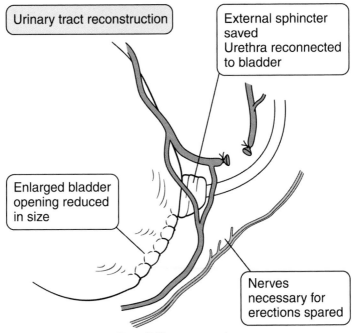

Urinary tract reconstruction

External sphincter saved
Urethra reconnected to bladder

Enlarged bladder opening reduced in size

Nerves necessary for erections spared

Figure D. The reconstruction.

If surgery is your choice, you should review the similarities and differences between the surgery types. There is little question that robotic surgery has become popular over the past few years. Despite the long-term outcomes of the types of surgeries being relatively similar, you should check with your surgeon about the latest differences in the types of surgery in terms of:

- Clinical outcomes, such as cancer control
- Erectile dysfunction and incontinence
- Hospital stay and recovery time
- Wound infection and scarring
- Blood loss and transfusions
- Pain

The nerves responsible for erections are located along each side of the prostate, run along the urethra, and come out into the pelvic area into the penis itself (see figure C). These nerves travel along with some blood vessels and collectively are called "neurovascular bundles" (there are 2 of them). If both nerves are damaged or removed during treatment, it is virtually impossible to have a natural erection without medication or a device (vacuum erection device or prosthesis). However, if only one nerve is damaged or removed, or if both nerves are spared, a natural erection or one that can be achieved with a pill is much more likely in the future. Before any cancer procedure always ask the doctor what the chances are that the nerves can be preserved. The goal of treatment is to remove all the cancer, so this may mean the doctor will not spare the nerves if it means there will still be cancer present. Still, learning about the fate of these nerves can help determine the type of penile rehabilitation that will be needed after treatment to allow a man and his partner to achieve the best sexual health outcome.

Radiation Therapy

In general, radiation is energy that is used in an attempt to destroy prostatic tissue while mostly avoiding injury to nearby organs and tissues. However, the bladder, rectum, and urethra are close to the prostate, so they may receive a small amount of radiation during treatment, potentially causing some side effects. Radiation therapy can be used in combination with androgen deprivation therapy (ADT), especially if cancer has spread beyond the prostate or the cancer is aggressive. Radiation therapy usually requires little or no hospital stay, and men can usually continue working and maintain their normal lives during the treatment. Radiation therapy comes in a variety of forms, including different types of external-beam radiation therapy (EBRT) and brachytherapy.

EBRT is delivered from an external source (outside the body). It is usually given in brief sessions (15 to 30 minutes), usually one session each day, 5 days a week, for 5 to 8 weeks. One type of EBRT is known as 3-Dimensional Conformal Radiation Therapy (3D-CRT). A computed tomography (CT scan) is used to create a 3-dimensional picture of the prostate and the surrounding areas so the radiation energy can be given only to the prostate gland. A customized treatment is designed for each patient before the radiation is delivered. Thus, 3D-CRT is an accurate delivery of radiation to the prostate target with the hope of more effective treatment and fewer side effects as compared to standard external-beam radiation therapy.

Intensity Modulated Radiation Therapy (IMRT) is a more sophisticated form of EBRT. Similar to 3D-CRT, a CT scan is used to outline the target and surrounding areas in the patient. The IMRT radiation dose can be changed across the opening of the beam, unlike other EBRTs where the intensity of the radiation beam is fairly constant during the procedure. Tomotherapy is the name of a specialized form of IMRT that allows the beam to hit the target from a variety of directions. CyberKnife (Stereotactic Radiosurgery) is another form of EBRT that also allows the tumor to be hit at different angles.

Image Guided Radiation Therapy (IGRT) is one of the newest technological advances in radiation treatment (a form of EBRT) for prostate cancer that also utilizes IMRT. Tumors and body parts move slightly within their body location, and IGRT attempts to resolve this concern. IGRT uses daily CT images and markers to pinpoint the exact location and size of the tumor and the surrounding healthy body tissues (bladder, penis, and rectum). Therefore, by using this procedure, radiation oncologists are better able to deliver higher and more precise doses of radiation at the tumor and minimize side effects.

SBRT (Stereotactic Body Radiation Therapy) is a type of EBRT that actually uses IGRT and is only given once a day for 15 to 30 minutes for approximately 5 days and then the patient is done with this treatment. The idea is to use higher and more precise radiation treatments, equating to what is given over many weeks with other types of EBRT. However, there is little long-term (10+ years) data on this treatment, so whether SBRT will be more or less effective as compared to other types of EBRT is not definitively known. Talk to your doctor about the latest research on SBRT if you are interested and ask him or her how the side effects compare with other types of EBRT. In fact, reviewing all the forms of EBRT with your doctor is extremely important because the field of radiation oncology is one that is rapidly changing.

Another specialized type of EBRT is neutron or proton radiation, which uses particles that have different qualities than the photons used in standard radiation. It also involves a good deal of pre-radiation target planning. Like other EBRTs, this treatment attempts to maximize the radiation dose that targets the cancer itself, but at the same time, it minimizes the amount that hits the healthy tissues. Some men with very aggressive tumors may receive a combination of neutrons or protons with a higher dose of another type of EBRT. There are currently only a few centers in the United States that offer neutrons or protons because it is very expensive technology. You should discuss with your doctor if it really works better than standard EBRT.

When a planning CT is used with any type of EBRT, small tattoos are placed on the patient's skin and the position of the prostate is measured from those markers. However, there are many different techniques used today to locate the exact position of the prostate before treatment. Some medical centers use ultrasound, others use CT or other imaging techniques, and still others insert seeds (small markers) into the prostate and take X-rays because the seeds can be seen on an X-ray to help locate the prostate. All of these techniques help to identify the precise location of the prostate because the prostate can actually move slightly over time. Exact location allows the treatment energy beam to hit the target better and avoid hitting noncancerous areas of the body.

Brachytherapy is a type of radiation delivered from inside the body. In this treatment, radioactive seeds or pellets are implanted in order to kill the surrounding tissue, including the cancer cells (figure E).Before the seeds are implanted in the prostate, a great deal of time is spent understanding exactly where the cancer is and the precise location of the prostate. There are different types of radioactive seeds that may be used, with Palladium-103 and Iodine-125 being the most common. The procedure takes one to several hours.

Temporary radioactive-seed implantation involves placing an intense radiation source directly in or around the cancer for a short period of time. Done under ultrasound guidance, 12 to 20 small, flexible plastic needles are inserted through the perineum and into the prostate (figure F). This procedure requires a short stay in the hospital.

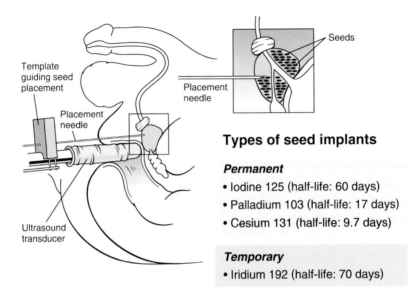

Template guiding seed placement

Placement needle

Placement needle

Ultrasound transducer

Placement needle

Seeds

Types of seed implants

Permanent

- Iodine 125 (half-life: 60 days)
- Palladium 103 (half-life: 17 days)
- Cesium 131 (half-life: 9.7 days)

Temporary

- Iridium 192 (half-life: 70 days)

Figure E. A side view of permanent radioactive-seed implantation performed under the guidance of transrectal ultrasound, or TRUS.

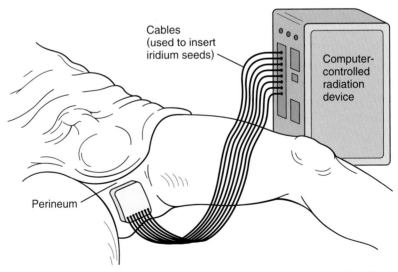

Cables (used to insert iridium seeds)

Computer-controlled radiation device

Perineum

Figure F. Temporary radioactive-seed implantation: Iridium seeds (also called "bars") are inserted and timed using a computer-controlled radiation device.

Some men who receive seed implants or external beam radiation are still potential candidates for receiving more radiation to the prostate if the cancer returns at some time. External-beam radiation may be used after seed implants, or vice versa, or more of the same type can be used in some patients. This may mean that some men are able to be treated with more seeds in the prostate if the cancer returns, or more external beam radiation to the area. While not a common option, it is still a potential option for some patients.

As you can tell from our quick discussion here, there are many different radiation treatment options and it is too complicated for anything other than a quick overview here. You should discuss in depth with your doctor if radiation might be the best course of treatment for your cancer, and if so, which type of radiation would be the best fit for you.

If you do opt for radiation treatment, a soft diet (low residue) is often recommended. The following chart gives you an overview of which foods are preferred and which are discouraged during treatment.

Dietary Group	Foods Encouraged	Foods Discouraged
Beverages	Milk/milk drinks, coffee.	Any alcoholic beverage.
Breads	Enriched white and light rye breads or rolls, crackers.	Breads or crackers with whole wheat flours, bran, or seeds.
Cereals	Cooked refined wheat, cooked fine-cut oatmeal.	Whole-grain cereals.
Desserts	Candies, cakes, gelatin, pie, ice cream, yogurt, pudding.	Coconut, seeds, nuts, tough skins.
Fats	Butter, margarine, cream, oil and vinegar salad dressing.	Mayonnaise, Italian or French salad dressing.
Meat, fish, eggs	Tender meats, eggs, cottage cheese, mild American cheese.	Highly seasoned meats, fish, or chicken.
Potatoes	Potatoes, macaroni, noodles.	Skin of potato, sweet potato, spaghetti, white rice wild or brown rice.
Soups soups	Cream or broth-based soups.	Others and spicy veggie.
Sugar/ sweets	Candy, honey, jelly, syrup.	Candy with fruits/nuts, seeds, skins.
Vegetables	Juices, canned/cooked tender veggies without seeds/skins.	All others.
Miscellaneous	Gravy, smooth peanut butter.	Relish, pepper, nuts, olives, salt pickles, popcorn, mustard, chili sauce, horseradish.

Reference: Liu L, Glicksman AS, Coachman N, Kuten A, Int J Radat Oncol Biol Phys. 1997; 38: 65-71.
Moyad, M, J Brachytherapy Intl. 2001; 17: 237-254

Cryosurgery

During cryosurgery (figure H), several super-cooled probes are inserted through the perineum (the area between the anus and scrotum) into different areas of the prostate. A warmer may also be used to reduce side effects. A trans-rectal ultra-sound probe (covered with a condom) is inserted into the rectum to help guide the procedure. When the probes are removed, each of the punctures requires a single suture, or

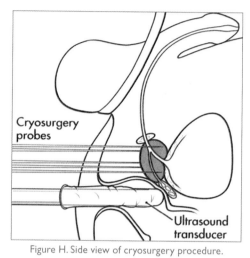

Figure H. Side view of cryosurgery procedure.

stitch, to close. Some doctors are also using cryosurgery today for men who have a rising PSA after radiation treatment.

Experimental Options For Localized Prostate Cancer (Non-FDA Approved)

Active Surveillance
(used to be known as "watchful waiting")

For a small number of patients, usually older men diagnosed with a non-aggressive prostate tumor that is small in size, an option may be to forego treatment for a period of time and monitor the situation carefully. This means you do not get any treatment for prostate cancer in the short term, but if the cancer shows signs that it is growing and may impact your life, then an effective treatment may be offered. There is no standard protocol for how to handle "active surveillance" patients, but I have summarized the most common procedures or methods used by the doctors who have researched this treatment. If this treatment may be an option for you, an important topic to discuss with your doctor is the anxiety of knowing you have an untreated cancer. Research shows that anxiety is the most common reason for discontinuing active surveillance. Although the disease may not have progressed, the uncertainty of not being treated when a patient knows that he has prostate cancer may not be acceptable to all patients.

What general requirements help a man qualify for Active Surveillance?
PSA Level of less than or equal to 10.
Gleason score equal to or less than 6.
Stage T1c to T2a.
Less than 3 biopsy samples with cancer & less than 50% of cancer in any one sample (however, this depends on age and other diseases the patient might have).
Older age.

What kind of schedule should be generally followed if you are on Active Surveillance?
DRE and PSA at least every 3 months initially for at least 2 years, then every 6 months if the PSA becomes stable. PSA, PSA doubling time, PSA density, free to total PSA and/or PSA velocity may all be calculated or determined while on active surveillance.
At least a 10-12 core/sample repeat biopsy after 1 year, and then every 1-3 years after this biopsy. Some doctors like to use imaging tests every so often, for example, transrectal ultrasound (TRUS), endorectal coil MRI, or another test that takes a picture of the prostate.
If the PSA doubling time is less than 2-3 years (in most cases, this should be based on at least 8 PSA measurements), there should be a discussion of potentially treating your cancer.
If on any biopsy the cancer has progressed to a Gleason 7 (4+3 in general) or higher, there should be a discussion to potentially treat your cancer.
Ask your doctor about the possibility of using the medications finasteride or dutasteride along with active surveillance for potential PSA and cancer size reduction. There are ongoing clinical trials with adding these drugs during active surveillance.

Reference: Dr. L. Klotz, 2010.

Note: There are several clinical trials right now that take men on active surveillance and treat them minimally with a pill, for example, dutasteride or finasteride or androgen deprivation, but these are all experimental studies with no long-term research.

High-Intensity Focused Ultrasound (HIFU)

This is considered an experimental treatment in the United States and it does not have long-term safety or effectiveness research. HIFU is an ultrasound beam that is focused at a fixed focal point (like a magnifying glass focusing sunlight on an object). It creates high energy that can destroy tissue. This means the temperature can become 80 to 100 degrees Celsius at the focused point, but not necessarily near the area or in the path of the beam. HIFU literally allows for "cooking" certain areas of the prostate from the outside inward. HIFU is a single outpatient procedure that generally uses a spinal anesthetic, and it has also been repeated in some cases if it fails the first time. It is being tested to potentially treat localized prostate cancer, and is also being tested for men who have their cancer return after conventional treatment. It is touted in some cases to have lower rates of incontinence and erectile dysfunction as compared to conventional treatment, but again this cannot be substantiated because there are no long-term data. Patients can usually return to work the next day. Immediately after HIFU, the prostate gland swells, which can cause bladder outlet obstruction and urinary retention. Therefore, a catheter is required for several weeks after the procedure. This catheter can be placed through the penis or through a small hole in the lower abdomen directly into the bladder (suprapubic catheter). As the swelling decreases after 3 to 4 weeks, the patient is usually able to urinate and empty his bladder. Still, there is a risk of incontinence, erectile dysfunction, risk of holes forming that can connect with different parts of the body (known as a "fistula"), and sloughing of dead tissue in the urine. Larger prostates can be a problem with HIFU because the heat can only go a certain distance in the prostate tissue. Androgen deprivation is used for larger prostates to first shrink the gland.

HIFU was approved by Health Canada as a potential treatment (available since January 2006), and some individuals have traveled there and other places to receive it. However, they have to pay out of pocket for the treatment, which can cost as much as $20–30,000 dollars per session. Regardless, this is an experimental procedure that needs more long-term research.

New Options And Thoughts About Advanced Prostate Cancer

Androgen Deprivation Treatment

One treatment for advanced and locally advanced cancer is androgen deprivation treatment (ADT), also known as LHRH treatment, which stops the production of testosterone by the body. Many prostate cancer cells need testosterone to grow, so suppressing testosterone can impede the progress of an advancing cancer.

Androgen deprivation treatment (ADT) can be accomplished in a number of ways:

- An LHRH injection can be given.
- An LHRH injection can be given along with an anti-androgen pill.
- The testicles can be surgically removed.

- An anti-androgen pill can be taken after the testicles have been removed.
- An anti-androgen pill can be taken.

LHRH injections are administered in the buttocks or abdomen. LHRH injections can be given every month, every three months, four months, six months, or even less frequently.

Is it best to give androgen deprivation treatment (ADT) immediately after a diagnosis of advanced or locally advanced prostate cancer, or is it preferable to wait until a man has symptoms? Some patients and doctors want to start ADT immediately, others favor a high PSA before treating, and others wait until there is clear evidence of advanced cancer from an imaging test, such as a bone scan. Each situation is different and should be discussed with your doctor.

Intermittent ADT (on and off treatment, also referred to as IADT) is being compared to continuous ADT in some very large clinical trials around the world right now. Since IADT is considered experimental right now, there are no absolute guidelines. However, IADT is usually administered by starting a man on ADT (LHRH injection plus an anti-androgen pill) for about 6 to 12 months, until the PSA is undetectable. The man is then taken off ADT and his testosterone is allowed to rise. When the PSA starts to rise and reaches a certain point, ADT is restarted and the cycle continues. Again, it is not known if this therapy produces similar, better, or worse results than continuous ADT, but it does seem to improve the quality of life in some areas, such as sexual side effects. Keep in mind that regardless of the type of ADT (continuous or IADT), at least 10 to 20 percent of men who remain on ADT for at least 1 to 2 years do not experience an increase in testosterone if the LHRH injections are stopped. In other words, the testosterone-making cells in your body stop making testosterone permanently following suppression.

What Happens if a Man No Longer Responds to ADT?

A review of all the options at this point is too extensive for any book. However, a quick overview of some options to help in the discussion with your doctor is provided in this section.

If your PSA continues to rise while receiving LHRH injection therapy (or another primary testosterone-lowering option such as surgery), there are several initial options, including adding an anti-androgen pill, or if you were also already on an anti-androgen pill, the doctor may stop it for several weeks and add another anti-androgen pill or simply move to other options, such as secondary hormonal treatment or chemotherapy. Keep in mind that, in general, the usual standard of care is to keep a man continuously on LHRH therapy during any other treatment from this point forward. There is evidence that there is still some benefit to be derived by staying on the LHRH therapy, including with chemotherapy or any other treatments.

Beyond LHRH Therapy

A chemotherapy medication, docetaxel, was the first medication ever approved for the extension of life for patients with hormone-refractory prostate cancer (HRPC, also called AIPC or CRPC). A patient is considered to have HRPC when his PSA level rises while he is on LHRH therapy. Docetaxel should always be discussed as an option for all patients who have HRPC.

Some of the more common side effects of docetaxel include low blood counts, fatigue, fluid retention, numbness in the arms and legs, and hair loss.

Since the approval of docetaxel, many other options have been developed and used for treating HRPC. The table below shows some of the many newer and older options. Each option has unique side effects, so talk to your doctor about the advantages and disadvantages.

Treatments for HRPC

Treatment	How do you take it?	How does it work?	Side Effects
Abiraterone (Zytiga®)	Daily pill usually taken with a daily steroid pill, can be used before or after chemotherapy.	Blocks the cancer cell's ability to to make its own testosterone to feed itself.	Increases in blood pressure, edema, and reduction in blood potassium levels.
Alpharadin	Intervenous (IV) radiopharmaceutical that reduces bone pain and improves survival.	Radioactive particle (alpha particle) goes to where cancer exists in the bone and delivers radiation directly at the cancer itself.	Anemia or a reduction in cells manufactured by the bone.
Anti-Androgen Addition (AAA)	Adding a first, second, or third type of hormonal pill, such as bicalutamide, enzalutamide, flutamide, or nilutamide.	Blocks the cancer cell's ability to use testosterone.	Can affect the liver, breast tenderness or growth, loss of libido, hot flashes, and even fatigue.
Anti-Androgen Withdrawal (AAW)	Stopping the anti-androgen pills, waiting over several	Over time, cancer cells begin to rely on some anti-androgen	No physical side effects, but if the response occurs it

Treatment	How do you take it?	How does it work?	Side Effects
Anti-Androgen Withdrawal (AAW) con't	weeks or months to see if PSA drops.	therapies, so removing it may effect a temporary control of cancer and PSA levels.	can be short.
Cabazitaxel (Jevtana®)	IV chemotherapy, usually given with a steroid drug every 3 weeks for those who no longer respond to docetaxel chemotherapy.	Blocks a specific part of the replication cycle of a cancer cell.	Multiple side effects that should be discussed with your doctor.
Denosumab (Xgeva®)	Injection given monthly or less frequently to prevent skeletal problems, such as bone fractures. May also be given every 6 months to men still receiving significant	A human monoclonal antibody that blocks a signal that would normally cause bone loss.	May cause fatigue, nausea, an injection site reaction, low levels of blood calcium, shortness of breath, and in rare cases osteonecrosis of

Treatments for HRPC con't

Treatment	How do you take it?	How does it work?	Side Effects
Denosumab (Xgeva®) con't	benefit on LHRH treatment(drug is known as Prolia® in this situation).		the jaw.
Docetaxel (Taxotere®)	IV chemotherapy, usually given with a steroid drug every 3 weeks.	Blocks the ability of fast growing cells to replicate.	Multiple side effects that should be discussed with your doctor.
MDV3100 (enzalutamide)	Daily pill, can be used after chemotherapy fails or may even be effective before chemotherapy (this is being tested).	Blocks the ability of testosterone to be used by the cancer cell.	Fatigue, gastrointestinal issues.
Sipuleucel-T (Provenge®)	IV immune enhancing treatment that does not reduce PSA levels. Used for asymptomatic metastati HRPC (before chemotherapy).	Immune cells from the patient are boosted and given back to the patient after 48 hours (3 treatments over 1 month).	Infusion-related short term/ temporary side effects such as chills, fever back pain, nausea, joint ache.

Treatments for HRPC con't

Treatments for HRPC con't			
Treatment	How do you take it?	How does it work?	Side Effects
Zoledronic Acid (Zometa®)	IV drug, given monthly or less often to prevent skeletal problems such as bone fractures.	Bisphosponate class of drugs that reduce bone loss by blocking the breakdown of bone itself by certain cells.	Side effects are similar to Denosumab.
Miscellaneous	Clinical trials and other secondary hormone treatments are available.	Talk to your doctor and go to www.clinicaltrials.gov for more info.	Usually low-cost, but these are not FDA approved.

Compassionate Use

Also known as an expanded access program, every patient with life-threatening cancer should know about this option. When a drug has not yet been approved by the US Food and Drug Administration for widespread use but it looks promising, patients may be able to access it by working through their doctor. Always inquire about the latest medications for compassionate use if you feel you are running out of options.

The Early/Expanded Access Program for Prostate Cancer Patients (EAPPCa) is a volunteer group made up of leading medical experts and patient advocates around the United States that came together for one cause—to ensure that any groundbreaking cancer drug that has completed a phase 3 trial and is waiting for FDA approval is accessible for no charge to the most desperate patients with the most advanced forms of cancer who are no longer responding to conventional treatments. EAPPCa has been instrumental in making sure patients have had access to several groundbreaking drugs, including recently MDV3100 (enazalutamide). If you feel that you are a patient needing to gain access to one of these future medications, please contact one of the national prostate cancer patient advocacy groups listed at the back of this book and inquire about any Early/Expanded Access Programs (EAP) that may be available or the latest information on the EAPPCa.

Preventing or Treating Side Effects

This chapter will quickly review the common and not-so-common side effects from some of the conventional prostate cancer treatments. We'll consider lifestyle changes, dietary supplements, and prescription medications that may help to alleviate or reduce the side effects.

Anemia (and other low blood cell counts)

What is it?

Blood, or more specifically, red blood cells are less able to carry oxygen to supply energy to cells throughout the body due either to a decrease in number of cells or a problem with the cells themselves. In rare cases, the anemia causes symptoms such as fatigue or shortness of breath.

Which prostate cancer treatment(s) are potentially responsible for this side effect?

Anemia usually happens with androgen deprivation therapy (ADT) and it occurs in the first few months of treatment in 90 percent of men. Testosterone is used in producing a hormone that helps maintain a normal red blood cell count, so a large reduction in testosterone is a common cause of this problem in patients having ADT. The type of anemia that usually occurs with ADT is known as a "normochromic normocytic" anemia, which simply means that the body is still producing normal red blood cells, but just not enough of them. Most men do not need treatment for this condition when it is related to ADT treatment, because the reduction in red blood cell count is usually only 10 percent. After several months, it either resolves itself or simply does not cause symptoms. Other types of anemia, such as microcytic anemia that is commonly caused from a dietary iron deficiency or macrocytic anemia that is commonly caused by a vitamin B12 or folic acid deficiency, are both uncommon with prostate cancer treatment. Other blood cells, such as white blood cells and platelets, can be reduced with certain types of medications, including chemotherapy.

How can it be prevented or treated?

Lifestyle Changes: Weight lifting or resistance exercise can help to reduce the risk of this condition, but patients with metastatic disease in their bones should get permission from their doctor. Lifting weights just two to three times a week helps to stimulate red blood cell production in men on ADT. Doctors do not usually want to give testosterone or another medication to improve this condition unless it is really needed.

Dietary Supplements: None recommended

Prescription Medications: Effective prescription medications (recombinant erythropoietin) that will help produce more red blood cells are always available if the anemia is severe. Additionally, a blood transfusion is an option.

Breast Pain And Enlargement
What is it?

Also known as gynecomastia, nipples of the breast become sensitive and painful and/or the amount of breast tissue in a man increases.

Which prostate cancer treatment(s) are responsible for this side effect?

Anti-androgen treatment (bicalutamide, flutamide, and nilutamide). The greater the dosage, the greater the chance of this side effect occurring during the course of treatment. Estrogen given to men can also cause this problem.

How can it be prevented or treated?

Lifestyle Changes: None

Dietary Supplements: None

Prescription Medications: There are two effective ways to prevent this from happening. The first is to take a daily anti-estrogen prescription pill, such as tamoxifen or any drug known as an "aromatase inhibitor." These work by blocking the ability of estrogen to stimulate the breast tissue in men. The only problem is that this pill usually has to be taken daily. The other effective preventive method is to receive a small dose of radiation to each breast (known as "prophylactic breast irradiation"). This takes very little time and usually only needs to be done one time. Finally, for men who have already experienced significant breast enlargement, the option of having a specialist remove some of this tissue has been successful.

Cholesterol Level Changes
What is it?

When the blood test for total cholesterol, LDL "bad cholesterol," or "triglycerides" increases, or HDL "good cholesterol" decreases.

Which prostate cancer treatment(s) are responsible for this side effect?

Anti-androgen pills (bicalutamide, for example) are responsible for lowering HDL when combined with LHRH treatment. Additionally, LHRH can increase triglycerides in some men. However, LHRH by itself can significantly increase HDL and this may come as a surprise to many health-care professionals and patients, but it has been a consistent finding in clinical trials. This actually makes sense, because high amounts of testosterone can lower HDL. Regardless, whether or not ADT impacts the risk of heart disease is not well known, but it reinforces the recommendation that prostate cancer patients need to know their cholesterol numbers as well as they know their PSA. This just makes sense in light of the fact that cardiovascular disease is the number one cause of death in men.

How can it be prevented or treated?

Lifestyle Changes: There are so many wonderful lifestyle changes that can change your cholesterol in a positive way and these are covered in chapters 1 and 2.

Dietary Supplements: Niacin is an excellent medication to improve HDL numbers in men who have lower numbers, and fish oil can reduce triglycerides in those with abnormally high numbers. However, keep in mind that all medications have some side effects, for example, hot flashes or liver problems with niacin and potentially a blood-thinning effect with high doses of fish oil. Talk to your doctor about the range of options available to improve your cholesterol and lower your heart disease risk.

Prescription Medications: Statin or cholesterol-lowering drug treatments are an option for men who cannot control their cholesterol through lifestyle changes. In addition, recent evidence suggests that these medications may reduce the aggressiveness and progression of prostate cancer. Even if they do not, at least they can reduce the risk of the leading cause of death in men.

A final note—blood pressure seems to be minimally impacted by ADT, unless someone gains a lot of weight—then it can go up. There is some concern that hormonal manipulation may also raise blood glucose or sugar levels and create a diabetic-like risk, but it is interesting that a recent study of men taking vitamin D supplements found a reduced risk of being diagnosed with diabetes while on ADT.

Cognitive Impairment
What is it?

Inability to remember some things and/or a feeling of mental fogginess or slowness.

Which prostate cancer treatment(s) are responsible for this side effect?

Some studies show that ADT or chemotherapy might cause this, but it is rare and other studies have shown no impact with these treatments. Regardless, if there is some concern at all, please talk to your doctor.

How can it be prevented or treated?

Lifestyle Changes: Mental exercises of all types help to keep the brain sharp (use it or lose it theory). Reading, crossword puzzles, card games, and any other activity that requires the brain to exercise itself, so to speak, can help. Aerobic exercise also helps to keep the human blood vessels clean and to allow good blood flow to the brain.

Dietary Supplements: There is some research to suggest that fish oil or omega-3 fatty acids (EPA and DHA) and vitamin D can help reduce the risk of cognitive impairment. There is very little research on the herbal product ginkgo biloba and it could thin your blood too much, so I do not recommend it.

Prescription Medications: There is some new preliminary research to suggest that low doses of estrogen may help prevent or treat this condition. Estrogen can also reduce bone loss in men on ADT, but it may increase the risk of a blood clot.

Depression & Mood Changes
What is it?

Feeling sad or listless, uninterested in life.

Which prostate cancer treatment(s) are responsible for this side effect?

In my opinion, just being diagnosed with cancer and going through any treatment can be a challenge to an individual physically and mentally. Therefore, it is important to discuss mental health before, during, and especially after prostate cancer treatment of any kind. Whether it is waiting for the next PSA or trying to get in a clinical trial or experiencing a new side effect, cancer can be stressful. Again, I am a big advocate of you and your partner evaluating your mental health during this time and seeking help if it is needed.

How can it be prevented or treated?

Lifestyle Changes: Heart Healthy = Mentally Healthy! Exercise, exercise, exercise! Research continues to show that it may prevent depression and, in those individuals on antidepressant medication, it may improve the efficacy of the treatment. Weight lifting or resistance exercise also seems to reduce the risk of depression.

Dietary Supplements: There are some dietary supplements that look interesting, such as SAM-e (S-adenosylmethionine) that has been combined with prescription medication in some instances. SAM-e has also demonstrated a pain-relieving benefit in arthritis, but the dosage (500–1,000 mg/day) or whether to even use it should be up to you and a trusted doctor. Omega-3 fatty acids or fish oil pills also have good research in this area. Of the omega-3 fatty acids in fish oil, EPA and DHA have the most evidence and are best when together in the same supplement or if there is more EPA as compared to DHA. Also, compare prices. These supplements can be expensive and most over-the-counter products have large price differences. There is an herbal product known as

"St. John's Wort" that is often recommended for depression and it may help. However, I strongly advise prostate cancer patients to stay away from this herbal product because it has been shown to reduce the effectiveness of many medications, including some cancer drugs.

Prescription Medications: Prescription medications are available and effective today. The most common medication classes are known as "SSRIs" and "SNRIs," and some of these same medications have also been shown to reduce hot flashes. Talk to your doctor about the options.

Erectile Dysfunction (ED) and/or Loss Of Libido
What is it?

ED is an inability to get or maintain an erection adequate enough for sexual activity or sexual intercourse, while a loss of libido simply means feeling uninterested in sexual activity.

Which prostate cancer treatment(s) are responsible for this side effect?

Most prostate cancer treatments have the ability to cause some degree of ED and/or libido problems. In general, localized prostate cancer treatment (surgery, radiation, cryotherapy) has traditionally been associated with some ED, and ADT or hormone manipulation has been associated with a loss of libido.

How can it be prevented or treated?

ED can take days, weeks, or months after prostate cancer

treatment to occur. Some doctors are encouraging patients to use a variety of ED treatment options (pills, pumps, etc.) soon after treatment to help reduce the risk of future ED problems (called penile rehabilitation). Talk to your doctor about this aggressive treatment option.

Lifestyle Changes: Heart Healthy = Erection Healthy. Exercise, blood pressure, cholesterol lowering, weight loss ... all can help to improve blood flow to the penis.

| DIETARY SUPPLEMENTS | | |
Type of Therapy	Advantages	Disadvantages
Panax ginseng (500-2,000 mg/day), has helped some men with ED	Cost effective dietary supplements.	Minimal research in prostate cancer patients.
MACA (1,500–3,000 mg/day)	Numerous small published clinical trials.	Minimal research on long-term safety.
L-arginine + pycnogenol (2,800 mg/day l-arginine aspartate and 80 mg/day pycnogenol)	May improve libido/ sex drive (including in LHRH patients).	Doses should be divided throughout the day.
L-citrulline (1,500 mg/day)		Other supplements can be very dangerous.
		Quality control issues.

PRESCRIPTION MEDICATION		
Type of Therapy	**Advantages**	**Disadvantages**
Oral medication phosphodiesterase inhibitors (also known as "PDE-5 inhibitors")	Pills taken by mouth. Effective for most men.	Not effective in patients who have had prostatectomy, unless some nerve-sparing approach was used. Side effects include headache, nasal congestion, and muscle and back pain. Should not be used in some patients. 15-60 minute wait for response. Cannot be taken with some medications. No impact on libido (sex drive).
		Can be expensive.

PRESCRIPTION MEDICATION con't		
Type of Therapy	Advantages	Disadvantages
Intra-urethral suppository (common doses available 125, 250, 500, and 1,000 mcg)	Small pellet placed in the urethra. Few systemic side effects. Effective in some men.	Can cause penile pain. Requires training. Can be expensive. Side effects include (rarely) painful and prolonged erection of more than 4 hours, fainting, dizziness.
Penile injection (multiple doses and options available, such as Bimix, Trimix and Quadmix, check with your doctor)	Highly effective. Few systemic side effects. Works in three to five minutes.	Requires injection. Requires office training. Can be expensive. Can cause penile pain. Can cause prolonged erection and penile scars or fibrosis.

| **PRESCRIPTION MEDICATION** con't | | |
Type of Therapy	Advantages	Disadvantages
Vacuum device	Least expensive. No systemic side effects. Effective in most patients. Battery-operated option now available.	Can cause numbness or bruising. Less "natural" erection. Trapped ejaculate. May be awkward to use.
Penile prosthesis	Highly effective. For men who have failed or are not satisfied with medical treatment of ED.	Small risk of infection. Requires anesthesia and surgery. May require replacement after many years of use.

Reference: University of California San Francisco Medical Center, *Managing Impotence—A Patient Guide*, N. Rahman, S. Rosenfeld, T. Lue, and P. Carroll, 2010;

Mulhall, JP. *Saving your sex life*, Hilton Publishing, Chicago, IL, 2008.

Moyad, M. *Dr. Moyad's Guide to Male Sexual Health*, Spry Publishing, 2012.

Fatigue

What is it?

A feeling of being tired most of the time.

Which prostate cancer treatment(s) are responsible for this side effect?

The most common causes are ADT, other hormonal manipulating drugs like anti-androgens, and chemotherapy. However, radiation therapy has also been associated with some degree of fatigue in some patients.

How can it be prevented or treated?

This side effect is being taken more seriously because it is becoming one of the most commonly reported problems with many cancer treatments. The good news is that there are now three different, but somewhat complementary, ways to prevent or reduce fatigue.

Lifestyle Changes: The first way is through a common lifestyle change—weight lifting. One of the most famous prostate cancer lifestyle studies ever done found that men on ADT who lifted weights about three times a week had an approximately 50 percent reduction in fatigue as compared to men who did not lift weights! Wow!

Dietary Supplements: Another method to potentially reduce fatigue is through a few dietary supplements. A large Mayo Clinic study recently showed that 1,000–2,000 mg/day of American ginseng (also known as "Panax quinquefolius") worked better than a placebo to reduce fatigue!

Also, past studies of L-carnitine (a compound made by every cell of the human body that helps improve energy levels) in similar and even higher doses may have helped. There is also a simple sugar known as "D-ribose" that when added to a beverage (1–2 teaspoons a day) has helped some patients with fatigue.

Prescription Medications: Last, but not least, the research on existing prescription drugs to reduce fatigue is interesting. Stimulant medications such as methylphenidate look promising, as do anemia drugs, if needed. Additionally, there is a medication taken in the morning known as "modafinil" or "armodafinil" that has provided some help for breast cancer and other cancer patients. Some doctors use it currently for prostate cancer patients with some success. However, more clinical trials are needed. Other stimulant medications with a good safety record are always being researched and may be available right now.

Hair changes and/or dry skin

What is it?

Hair growth on the head (yes, that is right), hair loss on the rest of the body (arms, legs), and skin that feels more rough or dry.

Which prostate cancer treatment(s) are responsible for this side effect?

ADT can cause hair growth on the head or a slowing of hair loss or a reduced risk of premature baldness. This is generally a side effect that does not get many complaints but needs to be explained. Testosterone is needed to express hair loss or baldness, so when testosterone is eliminated or reduced the human body responds by growing hair again (not a lot) or at least not allowing hair loss to occur. However, the situation is different for body hair. Most men in general lose head hair as they get older but gain more body hair, but the opposite occurs with ADT. Chemotherapy causes hair loss in general, especially on the head in some patients, but this side effect is reduced with some of the newer chemotherapy drugs.

Some men complain of dry skin issues when they are given ADT over a long period of time or certain other testosterone-changing medications. This seems to make sense if you think about menopause and women for a moment. When women lose estrogen over several years (menopause), they are more likely to experience dry skin. Men who have ADT experience a male menopause in about one to three months. So, it seems that dry skin can also be an issue that needs to be discussed.

How can it be prevented or treated?

No treatment is typically recommended for hair changes. There is no treatment needed for hair growth on the head and loss of body hair. Most men just want to know why it is happening. In terms of hair loss, there are wigs and medications that can help. However, in many cases it is temporary, so whether or not to treat it should be up to the individual experiencing it.

Lifestyle Changes: There are plenty of inexpensive and simple pieces of advice for preventing and treating dry skin. Dry air, cold air, indoor heating, friction, and even heavy clothing can make your skin dry, itchy, red, and it can crack easily. Long hot showers and baths are not a good idea unless you are with your significant other. Hot water removes the natural oils that the skin produces. ADT or not, as you get older your body produces less and less protective skin oil. Do not use the antibacterial, deodorant, or perfumed soaps, which can cause drying. Use a mild, moisturizing, and scent-free cleanser. Use warm rather than hot water. Keep the bathroom door closed to keep in the humidity, and do not dry your skin aggressively with a towel after the shower or bath because your skin needs to be a little wet when applying moisturizer.

Use moisturizer early and often, and place it throughout the house. A moisturizer right after a shower in the morning is perhaps the best way to protect your skin. Use a product with glycerin, petrolatum (Vasoline®), fatty acids (stearic acid, for example), ceramide, or cholesterol while your skin is still slightly damp. Reapply during the day as needed. If you use a facial and body moisturizer, as most people should, please use a broad-spectrum (UVA and UVB blocker) product with an SPF of at least 15 to 30.

Increase the humidity in your house. You can put a water-filled bowl near a radiator or heating vent, fill the bathtub, or just use a humidifier. Look for a device that has a humidistat, which is a control that automatically shuts off the device when the target humidity is reached.

Do not use an electric blanket unless it is really needed, because they remove moisture from the skin. Wear soft clothes and try to avoid wool and other rough fabrics. Try to wear cotton or silk next to your skin, and use an unscented fabric softener to avoid chemicals and perfumes that can cause excess drying. Use lip moisturizer with an SPF of 15 or more in it, or even petroleum jelly if you need it. You can treat cracked heels with moisturizers with lactic acid or urea and cotton-lined plastic or rubber gloves are a good way to go when cleaning dishes.

Dietary Supplements and Prescription Medications: None needed.

Hot flashes/hot flushes

What is it?

Sudden, at times dramatic, feeling of heat; may last seconds or minutes at a time and may occur regularly throughout the day or once in a while.

Which prostate cancer treatment(s) are responsible for this side effect?

Any treatment that reduces male hormone levels (ADT) can cause hot flashes, but the frequency and severity of hot flashes vary dramatically from one individual to another.

How can it be prevented or treated?

If you follow the steps in this section, you will become

more familiar with how serious your hot flashes are and whether or not they should be treated by conventional or alternative treatment, or if they should just be left alone. In hot flash clinical trials, most patients responded to some type of minimal intervention, but some patients can experience hot flashes that do not respond to simple lifestyle changes. For most mild to moderate hot flashes, a prescription drug is not needed, but for moderate to severe hot flashes, a prescription drug is usually needed. In the past, most men received prescription medical treatment for hot flashes, but recent clinical research suggests that only 20 to 30 percent of men need or ask for such medication. However, if you do need some help, prescription hot flash-reducing medications (especially progesterone pills and injections) work very well (Irani J, et al. Lancet Oncol, 2010; 11:147–154.). Researchers have learned from studies of women going through menopause that lifestyle changes may play a large role in the management of hot flashes. Before deciding with your doctor about the proper treatment for your hot flashes, you need to determine the frequency and severity of the hot flashes.

Using the rating scale that follows, you can assess the situation with your hot flashes. Just use the journal pages that follow to record your hot flash history for discussion with your doctor at your next visit. You may notice certain foods or activities that intensify the hot flashes and be able to make lifestyle changes that alleviate some of the occurrences.

Severity	Score	Length/ Duration	Observations
MILD Hot Flash	1 point	Less than 1 minute.	Warm & slightly uncomfortable, no perspiration.
MODERATE Hot Flash	2 points	Less than 5 minutes.	Warmth involving more of the body, perspiration, taking off some layers of clothing.
SEVERE Hot Flash	3 points	Greater than 5 minutes.	Burning warmth, disruption of normal life activities such as sleep or work, excessive perspiration, frequent thermostat changes in your house.
VERY SEVERE Hot Flash	4 points	Time is not an issue.	Complete disruption of normal activities to the point where it would make you consider discontinuing the androgen-deprivation treatment.

Personal Hot Flash Diary - Week 1

Date: _____

Day of the Week: _____

Mild = 1 point
Moderate = 2 points
Severe = 3 points
Very Severe = 4 points

Time of Day	Severity of Hot Flash (Mild, Moderate, Severe or Very Severe)	Points	Activity During Hot Flash

Number of daily hot flashes: _____

Average intensity: _____

Note on occurrences: _____

Personal Hot Flash Diary - Week 2

Date: _____

Day of the Week: _____

Mild = 1 point
Moderate = 2 points
Severe = 3 points
Very Severe = 4 points

Time of Day	Severity of Hot Flash (Mild, Moderate, Severe or Very Severe)	Points	Activity During Hot Flash

Number of daily hot flashes: _____

Average intensity: _____

Note on occurrences: _____

Lifestyle Changes: These remedies are my first choice, along with alternative medicines, for most men. By using the hot flash diary and some of the following low-cost lifestyle options, you may expect to see a 25 to 50 percent reduction overall in those annoying hot flashes. These methods are not sufficient for severe hot flashes so we'll discuss prescription alternatives later.

Lifestyle Change	Advantages & Disadvantages
Avoid hot beverages, spicy foods, and excess alcohol or caffeine.	Many foods and beverages can trigger hot flashes or make them worse. Your diary may help identify offenders for you.
Controlled, deep, slow abdominal breathing (6–8 breaths per minute) for at least 15 minutes twice daily (morning, midday and/or evening) or at the beginning of a hot flash.	Also known as "paced respiration," it has been shown to decrease blood pressure (temporarily), hot flashes, and the severity of a hot flash. However, this technique needs practice or it may need to be taught to you because it involves moving stomach muscles in and out.
Keeping a diary.	Diary-keeping for just 2 to 4 weeks can give you the best insight into what does and does not impact your hot flashes. Give it a try!

Lifestyle Change	Advantages & Disadvantages
Avoid smoking or breathing second-hand smoke.	Not only heart unhealthy, tobacco smoke makes hot flashes worse due to circulatory and temperature changes it produces in your body.
Low-impact daily exercise.	Exercise has been shown to reduce stress, improve mood, and it may reduce hot flashes. Use a fan or work out in a cool location.
Stress reduction (meditation, relaxation techniques, yoga, etc.).	Relaxation exercises can help with flashes and may also improve other areas of your life, such as sleep.
Use cooling methods— ice-cubes, cool beverages, fan reducing room temperature, opening a window, chilling pillows and/or pillow coverings.	If your body's core temperature increases slightly it can trigger a hot flash so it just makes sense to keep yourself a bit cooler.
Wear loose-fitting clothing and layer clothing.	Helps to keep your body's core temperature slightly lower, and prevents clothing from feeling constricting when a hot flash occurs. Layers allow you to easily shed clothing to regulate temperature shifts.

Complementary and Alternative Treatments

Along with the lifestyle changes discussed, these treatments are the best options for most men. It may be best to begin these prior to testosterone suppression, but you should check with your doctor before starting any treatment to be sure that they do not interfere with your cancer therapy. You would not want to consider more than one or two of these options at one time. As with the lifestyle changes, you might expect to see a 25 to 50 percent improvement using these treatments.

Complementary & Alternative Treatments	Advantages & Disadvantages
Acupuncture (1 to 2 times every week or two).	Few or no side effects, traditional needle and other forms of acupuncture have helped, not inexpensive.
Black Cohosh Pills (1 to 2 pills a day).	Moderate to expensive in price. Most research has been with women and shown it to work similar to a placebo.
Fish Oil Pills (at least 1200 mg a day total of EPA & DHA— the active ingredients).	Not expensive. New study shows it may reduce frequency of hot flashes. Also might reduce triglycerides and help with weight loss in men on LHRH. If you have a fish allergy, you can try one of the new algae-based omega-3 supplements.
Flaxseed Powder (2 to 3 tablespoons a day on foods or in beverages).	Cheap, high in fiber and omega-3 fatty acids, heart healthy, but lacks studies in men.

Complementary & Alternative Treatments	Advantages & Disadvantages
Magnesium Supplements (250 to 600 mg/day in a magnesium oxide).	Cheap and safe. However, most of the recent minimal research has been with women clinical trial currently using suffering from hot flashes during breast cancer treatment.
Red Clover Pills.	Moderate to expensive in price. Mixed research in men. May have side effects, and results are similar to a placebo.
Sage supplement or tea (100–200 mg/day supplement or 1 to 2 cups per day tea).	Helps with sweats. Needs more clinical evidence.
Sesame Seeds/Powder (2 to 3 tablespoons a day on foods or in beverages).	Cheap and safe, but most of the recent research has been done in the laboratory. More human research needed.
Soy Products/Protein (several servings a day or 20 to 40 grams of soy protein per day).	Cheap. Natural products (beans, powder, tofu) are heart healthy and may be more effective and healthy as compared to soy pills. As dosage is increased, so do gastrointestinal side effects.

Prescription Medications

These options are more effective as compared to lifestyle and complementary options in dealing with moderate to severe hot flashes. However, they can be expensive and all of them have side effects. If using them, always be sure to ask for generic equivalents to reduce your overall cost. On average, these treatments would reduce hot flash symptoms from 50 to 75 percent for severe sufferers.

Prescription Drugs	Advantages & Disadvantages
Clonidine Pills or Patches (0.05 mg twice a day or 0.1 mg once a day).	Least effective, but usually cheap in price.
Cyproterone Acetate (100 mg daily) or Chlormadinone pills.	Steroidal anti-androgens that are not available in some countries, including the US. Very effective (acts like progesterone), but cyproterone may have cardiovascular risks.
Estrogen Pills, Patches, and Injections (multiple dose options, usually less than 1 mg).	Very effective, usually cheap, and it reduces bone loss. However, some forms have serious cardiovascular and other potential risks (can cause blood clots, breast enlargement).

Prescription Drugs	Advantages & Disadvantages
Gabapentin Pills (average dose is 300 mg three times a day) or Pregabalin Pills (average dose is 75 mg twice daily).	Very effective, has a range of doses, but can cause sleepiness/drowsiness and dizziness.
Progesterone Pills, Injections (megesterol acetate at 20 to 40 mg a day, or medroxypro-gesterone acetate at 20 mg a day, or intra-muscular injection of 150-400 mg total of medroxyprogesterone acetate as needed).	Most effective, but may increase weight gain, reduce HDL ("good cholesterol"), and libido (sex drive).
SSRIs & SNRIs Pills Citalopram Desvenlafaxine Fluoxetine Paroxetine Sertraline Venlafaxine (multiple doses available but 75 mg a day of venlafaxine is one of the most popular).	Moderately to very effective, but has gastrointestinal (constipation) and sexual side effects. May cause weight gain, and some have cardiovascular issues. Recent large clinical trials showed that progesterone agents work better and seem to be safer. However, these medications may be more effective than progesterone for men undergoing cancer treatments who also have depression.

Incontinence/loss of urinary control

What is it?

This is a partial or complete loss of urinary control, which is also known as leakage and dribbling.

Which prostate cancer treatment(s) are responsible for this side effect?

Treatments for prostate cancer such as surgery, radiation, and cryosurgery are the more common causes, but this side effect has been reduced dramatically over the years. Today, only a small percentage of patients experience incontinence that requires a pad after treatment.

How can it be prevented or treated?

The prevention and treatment of incontinence is a large field of medicine and is beyond the scope of this book. There are many options available for prevention and treatment, including Kegel exercises (also called special perineal exercises) that can be done before and after treatment. These exercises involve strengthening the pelvic muscles by deliberately stopping and starting the urine flow. When not urinating, the same results can be achieved by tightening the muscles of the pelvis or buttocks. Regular practice of the Kegel exercises (talk to your doctor about how often) may reduce leakage or correct it permanently according to some doctors, but the results may vary from individual to individual. On average these exercises are repeated at least several times a day for several weeks or months. The opinions of doctors on the importance of these exercises and on other incontinence treatments after prostate treatment can vary significantly. Keep in mind that special undergarments, briefs, pads, pills, inserts (catheter), injections, biofeedback, and even surgery are all viable treatment options for mild to severe incontinence.

Muscle weakness/atrophy and musculoskeletal pain
What is it?
Loss of muscle/strength (also known as "sarcopenia") and/or pain in the muscle and/or joints.

Which prostate cancer treatment(s) are responsible for this side effect?
Any treatment that impacts or simply reduces male hormone levels (ADT) may cause muscle changes.

How can it be prevented or treated?
Lifestyle Changes: No surprise here! Weight lifting or resistance exercise and regular aerobic exercise of any type are the best ways to reduce the risk of muscle loss and weakness. Higher protein intakes may help, but talk to the nutritionist about how much you really need because extremely high protein intakes can cause abnormal changes in your kidneys, especially if you already have kidney issues.

Dietary Supplements: Recent research suggests that most men on ADT do not get the recommended daily intake of calcium, which is 1,200 mg per day. That, along with vitamin D, may help this problem. Only 1 to 2 pills of calcium carbonate per day are enough to meet your daily intake (see chapter 2). Recent research with vitamin D suggests that supplementation with an average of 800–1,000 IU may help reduce muscle atrophy and/or pain, but ideally it would be best to first get a vitamin D blood test (25-OH vitamin D test) before deciding with your doctor if you need more or less. A common dietary supplement that is used to improve muscle size and strength is creatine monohydrate powder, but the research is preliminary on this product. Most studies only use 5 grams or a teaspoon a day in a beverage for men who lift weights on a regular basis. I like to recommend minimal to moderate amino acid/whey protein powder supplementation that can be added to water. It should be around 100 calories per 8 ounces (around 20 grams of high-quality protein per serving). Recent research suggests it may work with weight lifting to reduce muscle loss and even help with weight loss at just 1 or 2 servings per day. This is very new and exciting research! As always, talk to your doctor about the latest research.

Prescription Medications: Some men inquire about growth hormone (GH) or other anabolic steroids to improve muscle mass, but there is a concern about long-term safety as they may stimulate cancer growth, cost, and the potentially lower quality of the muscle increase, despite a potential quantity increase. Talk to your doctor about these latest treatments. Over-the-counter pain medications can reduce muscle and joint pain discomfort when taken on a regular basis. Rarely, some men have had generalized body aches and pain (some call it "androgen deprivation syndrome") and some doctors have been able to control this problem with the use of low-dose prescription steroid medications.

Osteoporosis/bone loss

What is it?

Osteoporosis is a weakening of your bones that can lead to an increased risk of bone fracture.

There are no symptoms until a bone fracture occurs, so we need to consider how to prevent this from happening. First, we will discuss how bone loss is diagnosed. And then we will discuss how to prevent bone loss through lifestyle changes and what role calcium and vitamin D have in bone health.

An imaging (picture) test is used to help determine the status of your bone health. An imaging test usually takes a picture of one or several sites of the body and then your bones are compared to those of a 25- to 30-year-old male, the benchmark age range where individuals have the optimal bone health. If your bone or bones are similar to the benchmark, then this is considered normal. If your bones are a little less dense or a little weaker than the benchmark, this is called osteopenia. Osteoporosis is when your bones are much weaker than the benchmark. Finally, if you have already had a fracture and your bones are much weaker than a young person's, then this is called severe osteoporosis. The weaker your bones are compared to a young person's, and the more bone loss you have experienced, the more likely that you will experience a fracture in the future unless intervention occurs that reduces your risk of continued bone loss.

There are several devices available today to help your doctor determine the relative state of your bones. The three most common are compared in the following chart.

Tests	Advantages	Limitations
Dual-Energy X-ray Absorptiometry (DEXA)	Fairly inexpensive. Low radiation exposure. Rapid and easy to perform. Most multiple site-specific test for spine, hip, wrist. Recommended for most men.	Osteoarthritis of the lumbar spine and/or aortic calcifications falsely elevates measurement in older patients.
Heel Ultrasound (HUS)	Cheap, rapid, easy to perform in office setting. Low risk to patient. May assess initial risk for fracture.	Lacks overall sensitivity. Little known about accuracy of measurements over time. Not recommended for most men.
Quantitative Computerized Tomography (QCT)	Most sensitive method to detect osteoporosis of the spine. Recommended for some men when DEXA is not adequate.	Expensive. High-dose radiation exposure for patient.

I would make several general recommendations for your consideration when having a bone density screening done:

Recommendation 1: If possible, always have your imaging tests done at the same location, with the same machine, and same health-care professional to reduce error.

Recommendation 2: Always ask the health-care professional at the test site if the device is comparing your bones to those of a man or a woman. Ideally, you want them compared to those of a man.

Recommendation 3: Always ask for a copy of your results from the imaging tests and for a copy of the recommendations as a result of your test. Keep in mind that some individuals may get a test result that says that they have bones that are normal, osteopenic, and osteoporotic all at the same time because the multiple bones tested (hip, spine, and wrist) may be in differing conditions.

Recommendation 4: Make sure you understand the out-of-pocket and insurance-covered costs of the tests.

Recommendation 5: After you get your bone mineral density or osteoporosis test completed, use the web site http://www.shef. ac.uk/FRAX/ from the World Health Organization (WHO) to get another idea of your risk of bone fracture. You will need what is known as your hip (or femoral neck) "T-score" from your test results to complete the questionnaire on the site.

Which prostate cancer treatment(s) are responsible for this side effect?

Any treatment that impacts or simply reduces male hormone levels (ADT) may cause bone loss or weakness.

How can it be prevented or treated?

Lifestyle Changes: No surprises! Weight lifting or resistance exercise and regular aerobic exercise of any type are the best ways to reduce the risk of bone loss and weakness.

Dietary Supplements: Recent research suggests that most men on ADT do not get the recommended daily intake of calcium, which is 1,200 mg per day, and along with vitamin D may help this problem. Only 1 to 2 pills of a calcium supplement per day should be enough to meet your daily intake (see chapter 2 for more information on bone loss). Recent research with vitamin D suggests that supplementation with an average of 800–1,000 IU may help reduce bone loss, but ideally it would be best to first get a vitamin D blood test (25-OH vitamin D test) before deciding with your doctor if you need more or less.

Prescription Medications: The most commonly utilized pills or IV medications to prevent bone loss in prostate cancer patients are a class of drugs known as "bisphosphonates," such as alendronate, ibandronate, and pamidronate, and the most commonly used medication is an IV drug Zoledronic acid (Zometa®). These pills can be taken once a week, or in some cases once a month. Other options include prescription vitamin D injections and pills (cholecalciferol or calcitriol), which have to be taken regularly in the case of calcitriol. Research also suggests that a class of drugs known as selective estrogen receptor modulators (SERMs) may prevent bone loss, and the most commonly used drug is raloxifene, which has to be taken daily. Talk to your doctor about potential side effects (blood clots, etc.) of these medications.

There is some preliminary research that some of the osteoporosis drugs (especially bisphosphonates and Xgeva), which work so well to prevent bone loss, may also help to slow the progression of prostate cancer or block the ability of cancer to invade the bone. This is very preliminary. You should ask your doctor about this because these drugs also come with drawbacks and they may be overprescribed in some cases where just lifestyle changes and dietary supplements can prevent bone loss. For example, in a rare number of cases, they may increase the risk of serious jawbone issues (osteonecrosis of the jaw). I believe that any person who may go on the I.V. or oral drug form should first get clearance from a dentist to remove any suspicious areas of potential infection (for example, a partially impacted wisdom tooth). If the patient is already taking these drugs, he should see his dentist on a regular basis just for this reason alone.

There is also a new simple injectable monoclonal antibody (denosumab/Xgeva) the received FDA approval. It also seems to have these jaw issues. It will also be costly and has some potential drawbacks, so check with your doctor for the latest information on this drug.

Penis/scrotum shrinkage
(atrophy or genital atrophy)
What is it?

There are nerve bundles that run along the prostate and help to control erections. If any of them are injured or become less active, there is less of a stimulus or connection that goes to the penis and scrotum. This can result in a small change in length and/or width of the penis. Additionally, male hormone helps maintain the size of the genital area so when testosterone is reduced this can also potentially reduce the penis and scrotum area.

Which prostate cancer treatment(s) are responsible for this side effect?

Any treatment that may impact the nerves near the prostate and/or male hormone levels could potentially slightly impact penis size. Therefore, most prostate cancer treatments, from surgery to radiation to ADT, could potentially have this impact. Talk to your doctor about it and how it can be prevented.

How can it be prevented or treated?

Prescription Medications: The use it or lose it phenomenon of the human body can help prevent this problem. This means talking to your doctor about regularly using any of the erectile dysfunction treatment methods discussed earlier in this chapter in order to continue to maintain nerve stimulation and the length and width of the penis. Men have used pills, injections, pumps, and other methods to not only improve erectile function but to make sure that there is no reduction in size of the genital area. When the nerves have to be eliminated because of the cancer, talk to your doctor about what you can do about this condition.

Weight gain, belly fat/waist size increase
What is it?

Gain of non-muscle, fat and weight, especially in the belly or waist area.

Which prostate cancer treatment(s) are responsible for this side effect?

The most common causes are ADT and other hormonal manipulating drugs like anti-androgens.

How can it be prevented or treated?

Testosterone in men is needed to help keep metabolism moving, so anything that reduces testosterone or impacts testosterone can increase the risk for weight gain, especially in the area of the belly. And, as men gain weight, more triglycerides are stored in the belly area and the triglyceride part of the cholesterol test may increase.

Lifestyle Changes: Heart Healthy = Healthy Weight (see chapter 1). The best way to prevent weight gain is to reduce your total caloric intake and to exercise most days of the week for 30 to 60 minutes. This should be done before ADT begins ideally, because once a man gains a few inches or centimeters of belly fat it becomes even more difficult to get rid of it. Other studies of regular weight lifting have found that as a person increases their muscle mass their metabolic rate also increases. Therefore, regular aerobic exercise and weight lifting both help to keep fat off the belly. I like to know a man's waist circumference and pants size before beginning ADT, so that a goal can be set to maintain those measurements throughout treatment.

Consuming 20 to 30 grams of dietary fiber from food sources such as bran cereal and flaxseed has been shown to make you feel more full and help with weight loss (see Appendix One for more tips).

Dietary Supplements: Both fish oil and protein powder supplements helped improve weight loss when used with exercise. A study from Australia showed that fish oil (EPA and DHA) at 1 to 2 grams per day could help to reduce an additional several pounds or kilograms! Not dramatic, but not bad. Perhaps by reducing inflammation and triglycerides it may help to reduce weight, but taking too much fish oil can cause weight gain, so be careful. Other dietary supplements that help with weight loss have been a disappointment because they contain too many stimulants (caffeine) or other compounds that are heart unhealthy.

Prescription/Over the Counter Medications/Procedures: A study found that statin or cholesterol-lowering medication could reduce weight gain in men on ADT. There are several newer prescription medications that may help if needed. The best advice I can give you is that, regardless of what is offered to you for weight loss, a dietary supplement or older or newer prescription drug, always make sure that it is heart healthy and brain healthy before taking it. Some of the latest drugs that have run into problems have helped people lose weight but also increased the risk of depression!

Liposuction may reduce belly fat but has only been shown to be cosmetic, which means it has not been associated with heart-healthy changes (lowering of cholesterol, blood pressure). Some men inquire about growth hormone (GH) or other fad anabolic steroids, but there are some safety concerns. Although they may help increase muscle mass and thereby are cosmetically appealing, they are very expensive and have many more side effects as compared to lifestyle changes.

LHRH treatment checklist

As a final thought in the side affects chapter, I wanted to provide a checklist for patients undergoing LHRH therapy. The entries on the list are intended to be a combination of wellness tips for a patient in treatment and a reference to help with any side effects you may have. As we always advise, you should discuss the items on the list with your doctor so that he can recommend which tips might work well for your individual condition.

What to do during LHRH treatment	An option for me? YES or NO
Lift weights (upper and lower body) or do resistance exercise 2 to 3 times a week to prevent anemia, bone loss, fatigue, muscle loss, and weight gain.	
Do aerobic exercise for 30 minutes at least most days of the week to prevent bone loss, heart disease, weight gain, and to reduce the risk of depression.	
Consume a whey protein or another low calorie protein (about 100 calories/418 kj per serving with at least 20 grams of protein) or amino acid powder drink supplement to help control calories and maintain muscle.	
Take a calcium dietary supplement if you are not getting enough form your diet to help prevent bone loss.	
Take approximately 1000 IU (25 mcg) of vitamin D3 per day on average if a 25-OH vitamin D blood test determines that you really need to take more vitamin D.	
Once a year, take a DEXA test or another osteoporosis imaging test to determine if you have any bone loss.	
Eat a high-fiber cereal several times a week to promote weight loss. (For other caloric control tips, see Appendix One.)	

What to do during LHRH treatment	An option for me? YES or NO
Consider penile rehabilitation therapies (maintaining libido and penile length and width).	
Keep a hot flash diary for at least a week after treatment to track hot flashes for discussion with your doctor.	
Consume flaxseed powder for healthy cholesterol and hot flash reduction.	
Take a fish oil supplement (start with 1 to 2 pills a day) to reduce weight gain, triglycerides, and potentially hot flashes.	
Consider with your doctor taking a prescription progesterone pill or injection or another prescription if hot flashes cannot be alleviated by lifestyle and dietary means.	
Apply an spf 15 or greater body moisturizer to your skin after showering to prevent dry skin that can get worse with low or no testosterone.	
Keep your cholesterol, blood pressure, and blood sugar levels normal.	
Ask your doctor about the generic drug metformin for weight gain and blood sugar control issues if they are a problem.	

Appendices

Dr. Moyad's Waist-Healthy Tips

As we discussed in chapter one, deciding to maintain a healthy weight can be one of the most important choices that an individual can make for himself or herself. However, many men, and lots of women, struggle to make long-term changes in this area.

What I'd like you to realize is that weight control is an area where many small choices can contribute a great deal to achieving the result you want to accomplish. Your diet must fit your personality, but there are literally thousands of small tips that can be incorporated into your daily routine. Don't assume that you need to go on a very restrictive diet to see results. Studies show that most people who accomplish lifelong weight-loss goals do so by adopting a series of behavioral changes that fit their individual personality and needs.

To reduce your weight by one pound, you need to remove about 3,500 calories (14,654 kilojoules—kj) from your diet. You have to reduce your caloric intake by 500 to 750 calories (2,093 to 3,140 kj) a day to lose a pound or two a week. Even cutting out 100 calories a day for a year (419 kj)—fewer than half the calories of most candy bars—will result in the loss of 10 pounds. Double that to 200 calories a day for a year (837 kj)—still fewer calories than most candy or so-called protein bars—to lose 20 pounds. Add in some exercise and you've made a significant drop in your weight by just making small, sustainable changes. Now, doesn't that sound like a possibility?

In the chapter that follows, I've given you a whole list of suggested changes from A to Z. These are many of my favorite personal tips that help patients maintain their weight. Feel free to add in your own weight-loss tips to develop a plan that works well for you!

A

Alcohol

As we discussed in chapter one, any alcohol in excess is dangerous. The truth related to weight control is that alcohol is relatively high in calories, while it contains little if any nutritional value. This is why reducing alcohol has been a part of every diet program since the beginning of time! However, if you still want to enjoy a moderate serving of alcohol, there are beers that contain approximately 100 calories/419 kj (light beer). You can also drink a small glass of wine or use half the hard liquor on ice cubes or crushed ice and, again, you will cut your calories in half! Since it is certainly preferable to not drink any alcohol when you are trying to lose weight, try substituting herbal tea or sparkling water with a twist of fresh lime when you want to partake in your evening relaxation ritual.

Artificial Sweeteners

Artificial sweeteners or sugar substitutes can be your friend, but only when they replace actual sugar (known as sucrose, 50% fructose/50% glucose) with fewer or no calories. These sweeteners seem to constantly get bad press, but they do have a good long-term safety record and they have been shown to help with weight loss. Also, artificial sweeteners do not increase blood sugar levels. Stevia is my favorite sweetener because it is so natural and it tastes as good as sugar to me. Other artificial sweeteners include: acesulfame potassium, aspartame (NutraSweet®, Equal®), saccharin (Sweet 'n Low®), and sucralose (Splenda®).

You do not need more than 100 to 150 calories/419 to 628 kj of added sugar per day, and you do not need sugar-sweetened beverages and fruit juices. Do not worry about naturally occurring sugar in real fruit, milk, or plain yogurt. If a food contains little or no milk or fruit (natural sugars), the "sugars" number on the package's nutrition facts panel will tell you how much added sugar is in each serving. As we discussed, read those labels carefully!

Other natural sweetener types are also a potential option, but only if they also reduce calories because you use less to achieve the same sweet flavor. Agave nectar/syrup, honey, and brown rice syrup can be used in small portions (a half teaspoon or less) because they do have calories and increase blood sugar levels, but at least they give you an energy boost and taste good. People often worry about high-fructose corn syrup or HFCS (generally around 55% fructose/45% glucose). In reality, it has a similar fructose to glucose ratio (1:1) as other sweeteners (honey is 50% fructose/44%

glucose). The biggest concern should be the calories, so check those labels!

Sugar alcohols including mannitol, sorbitol, and xylitol are also used as sugar substitutes in some foods, but they can increase your blood sugar level. In some individuals, they can also cause gastrointestinal upset and diarrhea, so these may not be a good choice for some.

Bottom line for weight loss is that artificial sweeteners, when used properly, can reduce calories and will not raise your blood sugar levels.

B

Bagels

Bagels are high in calories and you should stay away from them unless you choose a "mini" bagel. It has fewer than 100 calories/419 kj as compared to a medium to large bagel that has a calorie count of 300 to 400 calories/1257 to 1676 kj. (That's without the cream cheese!) Remember what we said about increasing your fiber intake (page 24)? For more fiber to keep you full longer, look for 100% whole grain mini bagels. You can also add low-fat cheese (not cream cheese), salmon, or another source of lean protein.

Balsamic Vinegar

Balsamic vinegar comes from aged grapes and has 10 to 20 calories/42 to 84 kj per 1 to 2 tablespoons. It makes a great alternative to fatty salad dressings and works well as a marinade. Apple cider vinegar, made from pulverized apples, may be another vinegar to try. Start adding it to your diet in small doses as the acetic acid that it contains can irritate the stomach in higher doses. Hey, even apples themselves are low in calories, high in fiber, and require a lot of chewing, all of which translates into weight loss.

Beans, Beans (and lentils)

Beans are one of the largest natural sources of fiber in the world and are a good source of protein, too. When used in any breakfast, lunch, dinner, or soup, you are going to feel full on fewer calories. Yes, that means that a navy bean soup, soybeans, a lentil soup, or a vegetable chili is your friend—without the cheese, crackers and croutons on top, please. Mixing in chopped onions is not a problem. Try using sliced avocados on top for creamy texture instead of the cheese. Also, eat lower-sodium canned soup or homemade soup to keep blood pressure in check. Pureed beans also make good thickeners instead of creams in some soups and dips.

Be Bad Once In A While

Eat a high-calorie fast-food meal, drink, chips, or cookies—occasionally! Committing to losing weight long term means that it is okay to cheat once in a while so you don't feel deprived. Reach for your favorite delicious and decadent food or beverage or both! Remind yourself how good it feels to go low calorie on a regular basis and forgive yourself for an occasional indulgence.

Bowls & Plates

Research has shown that using smaller bowls and plates helps you feel more satisfied with smaller portion sizes. As we discussed, the ever-increasing size of portions makes it very hard to maintain a healthy weight. Using a smaller plate for your controlled portions can make them seem more balanced. Start using smaller-sized serving containers and watch how your desire for extra calories goes down.

Breadless Or Bunless

In many foods, such as a hamburger, a major chunk of calories comes from the bread or bun. Remove half the bread or bun and quickly omit 40 or 50 calories/167 to 209 kj while maintaining the same overall taste. Try to buy the bread or bun that has the highest amount of fiber and you will feel full faster on a smaller serving. There are new "thin" buns on the market under various brand names that are soft, flavorful, whole grain, contain no high-fructose corn syrup, and have fewer than 100 calories/419 kj per bun. Experiment with the toppings on your burger—omit the cheese and try salsa instead—and you'll realize even more calorie savings.

Breakfast (Part 1)

It is true that if you skip breakfast you end up just eating more calories at lunch or dinner. Never skip breakfast if you want to lose weight and waist. To save time on work and school days, prepare food ahead on the weekend. Cooked whole grains can be warmed in the microwave with a drizzle of honey or a few slices of banana for sweetness. I love brown rice, bulgur, and quinoa. Cooked low-fat turkey sausage is handy to heat, grab and go, or you can make a peanut butter sandwich with the 100-calorie thin buns. Focus on high fiber and protein to keep you satisfied throughout the day.

You can quickly add extra protein by including a portion of almonds, chicken breast, cheese, chickpeas, egg, lima beans, milk, oatmeal, peanut butter, salmon, tofu, turkey, whey protein beverage, or yogurt to your breakfast plans. Add a small amount of wheat germ (1 ounce is about 100 calories/419 kj and 8 grams of protein) to bran cereal or plain yogurt. You have not only added 3 to 4 grams of fiber and extra protein on top of the 13 to 15 grams of fiber in your bran cereal, but also the long list of nutrients that come from wheat germ would fill a children's multivitamin label. Be creative with your breakfast choices!

Breakfast (Part 2)

Cereals with the most fiber include All-Bran Buds® and Fiber One®. A quick word of caution, though, on the high fiber cereals, a serving is one-third cup! If you pull out your one third cup measure, you'll see that it would be easy to eat several times that much and wind up with a very high calorie breakfast. Measure carefully!

Check for oatmeal with at least 4 to 5 grams of fiber per serving and then boost the total by mixing in some bran cereal (double the fun). Pick the plain breakfast cereals (not the ones with added sugar such as yogurt bites or dried fruit) that have at least 13 or 14 grams of fiber per serving according to the nutritional label. For taste variety, you can mix a couple of high-fiber cereals in one bowl. Put some flaxseed or chia seed (both seeds are high in fiber and low in calories) or small fruits on the top, and you will feel full and regular.

Broiling, Boiling, Steaming, Baking, Roasting, Microwaving, Grilling, Braising, Stewing, Simmering, Stir-frying With A Little Oil

Okay, they don't all start with B, but these are the food preparation methods that make sense when trying to stay healthy and lose weight. Avoid frying, basting with fat, and cooking in fatty sauces and gravies.

Butter

Butter or butter substitute spreads are both fine as long as you use only 1 tablespoon per day. A tablespoon of butter is about 100 calories/419 kj and the lower, reduced fat, or flavored spreads are similar in calories or only about 25 calories//105 kj fewer per tablespoon. Use whichever you choose, but watch the serving size carefully! As we discussed, there are many tasty, healthy oils that are better nutritionally and can be substituted for butter in your diet, keeping similar serving size per day in mind.

C

Caffeine

Caffeine without calories is beneficial because it can increase metabolism and help reduce the muscle fatigue from exercise. Green tea (50 mg caffeine per cup), no-calorie coffee (150 to 175 mg caffeine per cup), and other teas or diet soda with caffeine are your best options. Sip a few ounces (too much can cause cramping) before, during, and right after exercise.

Candy Bars and Chocolate

The key here is portion size. If you just HAVE to have a sweet treat, the next time you buy a candy bar or chocolate, eat just half the portion you normally eat. You may satisfy your craving while getting only half the usual calories (100-200 calories/419-838 kj fewer with a similar amount of pleasure).

Canned or Packaged Soup

Soup that is broth-based is a well-known low-calorie food that you can eat on a regular basis without worrying about any weight gain. You may want to consume it before your regular meals to suppress your appetite. Watch the labels on soup cans to pick the ones that are low in sodium, unhealthy fats, and calories. In fact, most soup companies now sell "light" versions of their soups.

Charity

Events such as fun runs, bike races, swimming meets, or

just volunteering can be great ways to improve your mental and physical health and to help others. Participating every year in a cancer run or walk not only raises money for research, but it helps keep you slim and trim. Try and pick one or two of these events per year and do them with a friend(s).

Chili Peppers

Peppers such as habaneras (hottest), cayenne (very, very hot), serrano (very hot), jalapeños (moderately hot), or poblano (least hot, but hot) contain the ingredient capsaicin. The spicier the pepper, the more capsaicin it contains. These peppers have been shown to reduce hunger cravings. They also force you to eat more slowly and drink more water, both of which cause you to feel more full. Hot sauces, salsa (2 calories per teaspoon), and Cajun seasonings act in a somewhat similar way, giving you lots of options. Lots of flavor to your food without adding lots of calories!

Children's Portions

Eating children's size portions is one of my favorite methods to reduce calories at home and at the fast-food restaurants. You can save between 500 and 1,000 calories/2092-4184 kj on one fast-food stop by choosing the children's burger over the large adult meal. To increase your savings (and the nutritional benefit), try the apple wedges and milk instead of the fries and diet soda for more fiber, calcium, and longer-lasting fullness.

Chop and Slice, CHOP and Slice

By preparing your healthy foods in small pieces, it will force you to chew more when you eat one or two at a time. This sends messages to your brain that you are consuming more food than you really are and you will feel more full. However, a full stalk of celery or a whole carrot can still give you the same chewing satisfaction, giving you all the same end benefits.

Coffee without the Fancy Extras

While coffee itself has close to zero calories, thanks to all the creams and other items you can now add, coffee can be as high-calorie as a large dessert. If you need additives, ask for skim milk, add your own sweetener (try artificial sweetener, honey, or agave nectar), and a little cinnamon at the counter. It will taste indulgent while you save calories and money!

Cottage Cheese

Low-fat cottage cheese is your low-calorie friend. Cottage cheese is high in protein and is also healthy for your bones because it is high in calcium, all while having fewer than 100 calories/419 kj per serving. Other cheeses can also be good sources of protein, but watch portion size closely or the calories can add up.

Cough Drops

Similar to gum, sucking cough drops with menthol or

eucalyptus can be a good way to control your appetite, burn some calories, and keep your mouth occupied. And you thought you only needed these things when you had a cough?

Cravings

Cravings can be the Achilles' heel of most diet plans. They are often due to an urgent need for sweets or salt. Cravings occur at all times of the day, but especially in the late-day or nighttime hours. Being famished invites cravings to occur, so eating healthy, low-calorie snacks may help reduce cravings.

Rather than letting a craving derail your healthy resolution, when they strike eat some foods that are naturally sweet and not light (but still are low in calories). Focus on something that has healthy fats and protein to slow digestion and also some fiber to help make you feel more full. Pick any one of these or two together (or add some of your own) when those cravings hits you:

- pineapple slices, apple slices, and/or banana
- 1/4 cup of trail mix with almonds and dried fruit
- small piece of banana-walnut bread
- a handful of baked potato chips
- 2 or 3 squares of dark chocolate with high (70% or more) cocoa content
- 2 cups of air-popped popcorn
- edamame (soy beans) with sea salt
- teaspoon of peanut butter with some light or high-fiber crackers

- cheddar or caramel-flavored rice cakes
- a serving of nonfat Greek yogurt
- 1/3 cup of fiber-rich cereal
- 2 tablespoons of bean dip

D

Dips

Any dips should be less than 100 calories/419 kj and less than 100 mg of sodium per serving. Hummus, olive-roasted garlic salsa, creamy fat-free sour cream, and guacamole (also has lots of fiber) all make good dips for some fresh vegetables or high-fiber crackers. To be honest, for a treat, I like to dip baked chips in plain yogurt.

Diversify

Whether we're discussing the fruits and vegetables you eat or the exercise you do, diversification is the key. Many diet and exercise plans fail after several weeks due to boredom. Mix up the healthy foods you eat and the exercises you choose to help keep yourself interested and on track.

Dog Walking

Walking your favorite pet has been shown to help keep the weight off, because it forces you to get out there and walk daily or move on a regular basis. It is also a great way to meet other people. If you do not own a dog, you can offer to walk your neighbor's or friend's pet to get this weight-loss benefit!

E

Egg Whites and Yolks

Eggs are a great protein source, are low in calories, and are good for your eyesight! Try two boiled or poached eggs in the morning to make you feel full and energized during the day. Add some hot sauce (Tabasco or Sriracha chili sauce) to add to the full feeling. An egg is only about 75 calories/314 kj and 75% of those calories are in the yolk. If you're tempted to pass on the yolk, you should know that the eye-healthy compounds (lutein and zeaxanthin), vitamin D, choline for brain health, and almost half the protein all come from the egg yolk, so eat the whole thing. Regarding cholesterol and eggs, a couple of whole eggs a week do nothing to negatively impact your overall cholesterol level. In fact, a recent study showed that eggs may increase your good cholesterol (HDL), especially when on a statin drug, and that is a good thing.

Exercise

While it is true that you can lose weight without exercising, as we discussed earlier, exercise is closely associated with overall wellness and reduction of risk for many diseases. When we add in the additional benefits to your weight-control efforts and mood, exercise is a no-brainer. Pick a variety of activities to suit your tastes and get moving!

F

Fasting

Cut your total calories by 25% to 50% for a day every week or once every few days. Recent research has found that when you dramatically cut your caloric intake every other day or on a regular basis, despite eating a regular amount of calories on the other days, you can still lose plenty of weight and waist!

Fiber Is Your Friend

When comparing labels and calories, pick the food that is higher in fiber and it will help to reduce cravings. For example, nuts, seeds, beans, barley, whole-wheat spaghetti, or bran cereal has more fiber compared to plain spaghetti and sugary cereal. They make you feel full fast and help keep you regular as an added bonus.

Fish

Fish and other small seafood options such as shrimp are healthy, low-calorie additions to your diet. Grill, bake, broil, but do not fry it. If you like tuna in a can, make sure it is packed in water (not oil) for fewer calories. If you like sushi, try and eat the fish without the rice around it (sashimi) because you will save hundreds of calories on just 6 to 12 pieces.

Fish Oil Pills or Supplements

Just one to three fish oil pills a day has been shown to slow digestion, make you feel full, and help you lose weight. If you don't like the large pills, buy a children's flavored fish oil supplement and use 1 to 2 teaspoons a few hours before meals. As we discussed, you should consult with your doctor to see if you qualify for this supplement before starting any dosage.

Fruits and Especially Veggies

Eating fresh vegetables and fruit is a wonderful way to boost your nutrition while reducing your calories. They provide lots of chewing satisfaction and are low in calories as compared with similar amounts of other foods. Generally, make selections that are filled with the most water (least amount of simple sugar) to feel full and consume fewer calories. You cannot lose (but you might lose waist) with apples, oranges, strawberries, grapefruit, spinach, broccoli, and collard greens. How about an avocado, because it is loaded with healthy monounsaturated fat and fiber and can make you feel full? As a bonus, it has lutein to promote healthy eyesight and it has only 50 calories/209 kj per serving!

Fruit Juices

Fruit juices are reasonably high in calories, so try and skip them. When thinking of an apple, apple juice, and applesauce, the diet winner is the plain old apple. It contains the fiber, provides chewing satisfaction, and is low in calories. Keep this in mind next time someone tries to recommend a high-calorie juice for weight loss (no thanks). Carrot and other veggie juices are generally less than 50 calories/209 kj per serving. Not bad. So, veggie drinks are okay and usually contain some fiber. Aloe vera juice unsweetened is also less than 50 calories/209 kj.

G

Gluten Free

Foods or diet programs that are used by people who have an allergy to gluten (a protein in certain foods, such as wheat, rye, and barley) may be a healthy, low-calorie diet program that can be followed by individuals with and without a gluten allergy. Pick up a gluten-free diet guide at the bookstore and see how many healthy low-calorie options exist. A diabetic diet book may also provide very healthy low-calorie options that are good for diabetics and nondiabetics alike.

Gum Chewing

Chewing a piece of gum actually burns calories and keeps your mind off of eating, so pick a no-calorie, sugar-free gum and chew, chew, chew ... to lose, lose, lose.

Grilling

We mentioned grilling earlier as a low-calorie preparation option. Grilling steak or chicken uses less oil compared to pan-frying. Use that grill, season with low-calorie spices and lemon, and it should help in the battle of the bulge.

H

Half Portion

This relates to portion size that we discussed earlier. When you are not in control of your own portion size, such as when eating at a restaurant or a family event, plan to eat half of what is being served. At a restaurant, you can ask for a "to-go" box when you order and immediately put half the food in the box as soon as the server brings it. You will still feel the satisfaction of clearing your plate! Over time, this can result in significant weight loss and you will recognize that most of us consume too many calories. Truth is that people from Asia and some Mediterranean countries actually consume about 50% fewer calories as compared to many Americans! So, try this for a few days and see how you do.

Honey

Honey is a low-calorie, natural sweetener option. Just a teaspoon or two per day can satisfy your sugar cravings. Skip that sugary snack or dessert and use honey to boost energy and immunity. A recent large clinical trial also shows that it can even help you recover faster from an illness and sleep better.

K

Kale

Kale probably qualifies as a miracle food. It can be chopped up and used with a small amount of olive oil, in soups, salads, stir-fries, and breakfast omelets. It is fibrous, low in calories, and loaded with all sorts of healthy nutrients, such as calcium.

L

Lean

Meats that are lean, such as certain cuts of chicken, pork, turkey, and beef, are always better than non-lean choices. Look for meats that are more than 90% lean because they are high in protein and have fewer calories.

Lemonize or Limeonize

I'm not sure they are words, but still worth considering. Squeeze lemon or lime on anything and everything that usually has high-calorie sauces or dressings, for example, salads. You will get the entire flavor and none of the calories!

M

Medications or Supplements

Medicines or supplements that help lower cholesterol (especially triglycerides) may also help with weight loss. A recent study has found that keeping your numbers low may reduce or maintain weight by limiting the amount of fat (triglyceride) that is stored deep in the body. These medications are not prescribed for weight loss but using them compliantly if you need them may provide that added benefit.

Milk

Keep it skim to stay trim! An 8-ounce serving of whole milk (160 calories/669 kj) has double the calories of skim, soy, or rice milk (80 calories each/335 kj). Just going from 0.5% to 1% to 2% adds another 10, 20, and 40 calories per cup as compared to skim milk. However, it is important to drink milk, so if you don't like the taste of skim milk, choose the lowest-fat milk that satisfies your taste requirements. You may want to try one of the new novel milks, for example, almond milk, which is about 40 to 60 calories per serving.

Muscle Protein or Milk/Whey Protein

Protein drinks now come in 100 calorie/419 kj or less per servings. They provide a substantial quantity (10 to 20 grams) of high-quality protein. They can be purchased as powder that you mix with water or they now come already packaged and ready to drink, so it helps you feel full more quickly.

Mustard

With no calories, mustard can be a good alternative to mayonnaise or another high-calorie condiment on your sandwich or sub. If you miss the creamy texture, you can spread on mashed avocado and get a bonus of healthy monounsaturated fat and other nutrients!

N

Nuts

While nuts are very nutritious, they can also be high in calories so we need to include them carefully in our weight-conscious diet. Pick a low-calorie nut such as two handfuls of pistachios for only 160 calories/669 kj. Pistachios are one of the lowest-calorie nuts. You should remove the shell yourself because that extends the time taken to eat your snack. Or just eat one small handful of your favorite nuts. Cocoa powder-coated almonds are delicious and they can satisfy your chocolate craving, too.

O

Oils, Oils, Oils

When considering weight loss, oils equal calories. As we advised with butter, they should be used in very controlled quantities. Always remember that even the healthy oils such as olive, safflower, and canola, are all 120 calories/ 502 kj per tablespoon. As an alternative, use an oil spray that has few or no calories when cooking, or use these oils as a substitute for something that may have even more calories.

Omega-3 Fatty Acids

Omega-3 fatty acids are healthy fats found in flaxseed , chia seeds, and fish. We discussed the health benefits of Omega-3 fatty acids on page 19, but an added benefit to dieters is that they help you to feel full. Both flaxseeds and chia seeds are rich in fiber, so put regular flaxseed, golden flaxseed, hemp seeds or oil (yes, these are legal and safe), or chia seeds on cereal or in a salad and your colon and waistline will thank you!

P

Pasta

Whole-wheat or whole-grain pastas contain as much protein and more fiber than regular white pasta. They are filling and can be served with a variety of delicious toppings, such as steamed vegetables or chicken breast to make a meal. Try buckwheat pasta if you get a chance because it is one of the best pastas in terms of protein and the potential for weight loss. Be sure to keep your pasta serving size to one healthy cup and avoid high-fat accompaniments such as meatballs or sausage.

Pickles

Pickles make a great crunchy, low-calorie snack, but be sure to pick the low-sodium varieties to keep them heart-healthy.

Pizza

By ordering "thin crust" and "light cheese" with your favorite veggies, you can have pizza and still mind your waistline. Two pieces of thin-crust veggie pizza have at least 500 fewer calories/2092 kj as compared to two deep-dish or regular slices! Broccoli, peppers, and mushrooms on your thin crust pizza will not add many calories and will make you feel more full. Ask for whole-wheat crust if it is available.

Popcorn

From the microwave or air-popped, popcorn can be a great snack that is fat-free. It can have as many as 700 fewer calories/2929 kj than movie-theater popcorn. Add some sprinkles of fresh brewer's yeast on top of the popcorn (instead of butter), and you now have yourself a nutritious, low-calorie, tasty snack.

Pomegranate Seeds

Given the choice on pomegranate—the entire fruit, the juice, or the seeds—the seeds are arguably the best weight-loss option. They are not only low in calories but they are also high in fiber and make a great snack.

Portion Control

Using mental pictures to help you judge portion size is a simple way to cut calories and lose weight. See if some of the images below help you stick to consuming only one portion of these foods at any meal.

Cheese slice = 1 playing card

Fish = a checkbook

Meat = a deck of cards or a bar of soap

Pasta = a tennis ball

Peanut butter or another spread on bread = a golf ball

Potato = a computer mouse

Rice = scoop of ice cream

Processed Food

Generally speaking, foods in their natural state tend to be lower in calories and higher in fiber. Picking natural or minimally processed choices may help reduce your weight while improving your nutrition. See how many things you consume from the first column below.

Natural Product Unprocessed (The right choice)	Minimally Processed Product (Okay in some cases)	Highly Processed Product (Less is preferred)
Apple has fiber and potassium, low in calories.	Applesauce healthy still, but a lot less nutritious and filling.	Apple toaster pastry.
Artichoke loaded with fiber.	Artichoke hearts.	Artichoke dip high in calories and sodium.
Beef—grass fed higher in nutrients and lower in fat.	Beef—grain fed.	Beef—frozen patties.
Brown rice has its fiber-rich layers.	White rice.	Instant rice—flavored.
Carrots lots of chewing enjoyment.	Baby carrots Healthy, but stripped of fiber.	Frozen flavored/glazed carrots.
Chicken drumstick/ breast with skin removed.	Sliced chicken in deli.	Chicken nuggets.
Corn on the cob	Frozen corn.	Corn chips.
Eggs—pasture-raised more nutrients and omega-3.	Eggs—fortified omega-3.	Egg beaters.
Figs.	Fig preserves.	Fig sandwich cookies.
Garlic.	Minced garlic in jar.	Garlic bottled marinade.
Grapes.	Raisins watch the calories when combined with trail mixes.	Wine watch the calories.

Natural Product Unprocessed (The right choice)	Minimally Processed Product (Okay in some cases)	Highly Processed Product (Less is preferred)
Ham—Heritage less hormones.	Ham slices.	Bologna.
Orange has fiber.	Orange juice.	Orange drink.
Peach.	Canned peaches in juice.	Canned peaches in syrup.
Peanuts.	Peanut butter spread (natural).	Peanut butter in a jar.
Pineapple.	Canned pineapple	Pineapple cocktail cup.
Soup—homemade less sodium and more flavor.	Canned soup.	Dehydrated soup mixture.
Soybeans— whole/edamame low in calories, high fiber.	Tofu.	Frozen veggie burgers, hot dogs, or soy cheese.
Spinach.	Bagged and prewashed spinach.	Frozen creamed spinach.
Strawberry.	Strawberry jam/ preserves.	Strawberry gelatin
Turkey (whole).	Sliced turkey free of most fillers and nitrates.	Turkey meatball.
Whole-grain bread	Wheat bread.	White bread—fortified.
Whole-wheat pasta high in fiber and antioxidants.	Regular pasta.	Instant noodles/ramen.
Yogurt—plain flavor it yourself with fruit or honey.	Flavored yogurt.	Yogurt flavored drink.

Protein

Protein should come from a high-quality food (beef, chicken, eggs, fish, beans) or beverage (whey powder or soy protein) because you will pay less, get a higher-quality protein, and will not get all the added calories as compared to getting your protein from a protein bar. The rule we discussed above on choosing less-processed foods definitely applies here.

Q

Quinoa

If you haven't heard of quinoa yet (pronounced kin-wa), give it a try. This small grain is higher in quality protein as compared to other grains, such as rice, millet, and wheat. Add in that it is low in calories, high in fiber, and gluten-free, and you'll see why you may want to add it to your diet. It can be substituted for any grain in most recipes, mixed with honey for breakfast, used as a side with any lunch or dinner, or used in soups, salads, and cold dishes. It takes only 10 to 15 minutes to prepare.

S

Salad Toppings

The things you pile on top of your lettuce can take a salad from a natural, nutritious meal to a high-calorie diet buster. If you think of bacon, cheeses, dried fruits, croutons, creamy dressings, and caramelized nuts, you'll see what I mean. To keep your salad on track as a healthy meal, instead add low-calorie veggies such as cucumbers, mushrooms, bell peppers, and onions. Try some green peas or another low-cal option—chickpeas. Then, either use half the dressing you would normally use or a low-calorie dressing such as balsamic vinegar. Experiment with another vinegar-based low-calorie dressing, such as mustard vinaigrette, or try some of the spray salad dressings that add lots of flavor without the fat and calories of regular dressings.

Saturated Fat

Whenever you are comparing labels from similar products, such as milk, meat, chips, fast foods, make sure you pick the item with less saturated fat because this will usually result in fewer calories. It pays to get in the habit of reviewing nutritional labels carefully, as many times a slight change in choices can result in major calorie savings.

Sea Salt

Sea salt has more flavor than regular salt, which will allow you to use less in your food. As we discussed, it is important to monitor your total sodium intake, some of which comes from salt you add to your food. Be sure to also monitor nutritional labels to find the sodium contained within processed foods. That sodium can amount to 80% of your total intake every day.

Seeds

Generally speaking, seeds are low in calories and high in

protein, which can help you reduce your appetite. Sunflower, pumpkin, sesame, flaxseed, and chia seeds are also heart-healthy, containing a high amount of healthy fat and a low amount of unhealthy fat.

Skinless

When you remove the skin from poultry, you are removing loads of calories, as much as 40% to 50% of the fat, and the largest source of cholesterol. And, in some cases, such as turkey, the lighter the meat the fewer the calories!

Sleep

Suppose I told you that you could sleep more and weigh less? Research has shown that individuals who do not get enough sleep eat more calories during the day. Going with less sleep allows you to snack and drink more, and it increases stress compounds in your body that can cause weight gain. Get the proper rest and save on calories, too.

Slow and Stop

These two words are important to remember when you are eating. When you eat slowly, your brain has time to re-alize you have really had enough to eat and it will send a message to your body, stopping you from overeating. Also, eating slowly will allow you to fully enjoy the smells and tastes of your food. A final tip, STOP eating and drinking immediately when you feel your hunger or thirst begin to subside. Don't wait until you feel full because, by the time your body recognizes it is full, you've actually overeaten.

Smoothie

Smoothies can be a good choice or a really poor choice. If you purchase one out, it may average between 500 and 1,000 calories/ 2092-4184 kj. To keep it healthy, create your own using fat-free yogurt, skim milk, and your favorite fruit. Another option, make yourself a powdered whey protein drink using 8 ounces/236 ml of water for around 100 calories/419 kj. If you feel adventurous, try a no-calorie or low-calorie shot or drink from the health food store, such as a veggie or aloe vera unsweetened juice or simply wheatgrass.

Snack

Snacking often on low-calorie veggies, low-calorie fruit, rice cakes, or other low-calorie treats helps to keep your hunger cravings from getting out of control. Research shows that individuals who snack sensibly 4 to 5 times a day tend to eat less at their regular meals and lose weight.

Socialize

Studies show that humans are more likely to feel better and stick to an exercise program when it involves others. And, if you surround yourself with individuals who have similar activity and weight levels to your goal, you are more likely to be successful in achieving that goal. This is why support groups are helpful. Whether or not you are inclined to work out with others, try picking an organized class at least once a week and go with a friend. It will keep you motivated, committed, and help you lose weight and waist along with the other people in the class you are attending.

Sparking Water

Sparkling or carbonated water tends to make you feel a little full, so drinking a glass before or with a meal may reduce your food consumption. This is another good one to lime-onize or lemonize!

Spices

Spices add a bonus of flavor to your foods without adding extra calories. Seven super spices may also have added health benefits, namely: cinnamon, ginger, oregano, red pepper, rosemary, thyme, and tumeric. Spice up your food and enjoy!

Spray

Homemade or purchased food sprays are a great way to get fewer calories. A butter, oil, or salad dressing spray allows you to spritz on the flavor and texture of the high-calorie product with almost no calories. Use cooking sprays to prepare your food without adding butter or oil to the pan or grill.

Stairs

Skip the elevator, escalator, or moving sidewalk and you will find yourself burning more calories.

Steamed Veggies

Order them when you go out to eat because they will make you feel full and they have hundreds of calories fewer than the fries and onion rings that you might have normally ordered. Steamed veggies will always be a better choice compared to any fried product. Sprinkle them with a no-salt seasoning product to add a little zip.

Stress

Stress causes weight gain and increases the risk of other health problems. Whether you like to play golf, meditate, do yoga, breathe more deeply, walk, bike, or simply socialize, reducing your stress is always a good choice. Experiment a bit to find your own personal cure for stress.

Sugar

Avoid adding extra sugar to foods whenever possible. As advised earlier, you may want to try no-calorie or low-calorie substitutes to sugar, such as stevia, agave, or honey. Adding fresh fruit will often satisfy your need for something sweet.

T

Tea

A cup of warm or iced tea is a soothing and filling beverage. Green, oolong, and black have caffeine while most herbal and rooibos tea has little or no caffeine and oxalate (good for those with a past history of kidney stones). Tea should be part of any healthy weight-control program.

Television

Watching television is time spent sitting instead of being involved in a more active pursuit. And, as we all know, it can lead to more snacking! Reducing your TV time can contribute to that 500 calories/2092 kj a day reduction goal.

V

Vegetarian

Thinking vegetarian when you go to a fast-food restaurant or shopping for food can be a great way to cut calories and increase nutrition. The vegetarian option at fast-food restaurants, such as sub shops or pizza places, is usually the low- or lowest-calorie choice. Be sure that you watch the toppings you add on your sub though. Picking mustard instead of mayonnaise can help keep that calorie count low. Vegetarian choices at the grocery store can be used to boost nutrition while helping you maintain your waistline. Did you know that some people call themselves "flexitarian" when they enjoy meat occasionally? They choose to use meat more as a flavor enhancer or condiment, and they eat mostly plant-based foods?

Veggies

Vegetables are one of the few foods that generally follow the "more is better" philosophy. They are loaded with fiber and, in general, low in calories. A few starchy vegetables, such as carrots and potatoes, are higher in calories and should be included in your diet in moderation, but most vegetables are great for unlimited munching. For example, cucumbers, celery, and mushrooms have virtually no calories but are filled with healthy antioxidants.

Vitamin D

Taking a 1000 IU (25 mcg) supplement of vitamin D a day may help you reduce belly fat by producing anti-stress compounds in your body. Vitamin D is discussed in more depth earlier, but it is an important nutrient to consider for your health in general.

W

Water

Similar to what was discussed in sparkling water, drinking water before or with your meals can help you to feel full and eat fewer calories. Did you also know that the colder the water, the more your body has to increase metabolism to make sure the temperature of the water becomes the same as your body temperature, which can help you even more with a little weight loss.

Weight Lifting

Weight lifting is a great way to reduce your waist size (even without cutting calories) and it also reduces your risk of muscle loss as you get older. It is one of the best ways to increase your metabolism, so it becomes easier to burn calories. Muscle burns more calories compared to fat, even when you are sitting or sleeping! One of the smartest ways to lose some waist as you get older is to lift weights (upper and lower body) 2 to 3 times a week.

Whey Protein Concentrate

Whey protein concentrate, isolate, and even hydrolysate powder and flavored products (such as strawberry and chocolate) can be added to a glass of water (15–30 grams) and should be about 100 calories/419 kj or less per serving. Drinking one of these flavored drinks a day can make you feel more full. It has been shown to help with weight loss and to help prevent muscle loss, along with diet and exercise, of course.

Whole Grain

Whole- or multi-grain foods, such as breads, pastas, and brown rice, are a quick way to increase fiber and feel more full. Look for the "whole grain" or "whole wheat" or "multi-grain" labels next time you are at the local grocery store. Make sure it is 100% whole grain or that whole grain is the first item in the list of ingredients. This tells you that there is more than just a sprinkle of whole grains, which is sometimes used as a marketing trick. These products should have about the same calories and more fiber compared to the similar alternative non-whole grain or non-wheat products.

Y

Yogurt

Plain, not flavored, yogurt is a simple low-calorie way to keep your digestive tract healthy as it contains friendly bacteria that can improve your metabolism. You may even want to use it instead of heavy cream in a favorite baking recipe such as banana bread or as a substitute for sour cream.

Z

Zero

Zero calories are always good, but remember that you can reach your weight-loss goals by making a series of small steps and choices to improve your diet and boost your activity. You've read through my favorite tips, so now get creative and come up with some that will work well for you. Then, set your sights on your goal and get started!

A Final Note ...

Dealing with cancer can be very stressful and confusing both for patients and their families. It helps to continue to educate yourself so that your discussions with your doctor are productive and together you develop a treatment plan that best matches your individual needs and situation. No one resource or book can provide all the information on a given topic, but hopefully we've given you an overview with this publication. Remember to make a list of questions before your visits to your healthcare provider so that you don't forget to ask certain things that are important to your well being.

There are a host of resources available to patients and caregivers. I've listed just a few here that may be of particular use. Don't forget, in combating an illness, knowledge can be your best ally!

Advocacy And Support Organizations
Alliance for Prostate Cancer Prevention
> www.apcap.org

American Cancer Society
> www.cancer.org

American Society of Clinical Oncology
> www.asco.org

American Urological Association
> www.auanet.org

CancerCare
> www.cancercare.org

Foundation for Cancer Research and Education
> www.cancer-foundation.org

HRPCa.org.
> www.hrpca.org

MaleCare
www.malecare.org
Man to Man, local groups of the American Cancer Society
www.cancer.org/treatment/supportprogramsservices/index
National Alliance of State Prostate Cancer Coalitions
www.naspcc.org
National Comprehensive Cancer Network
www.nccn.org
Patient Advocates for Advanced Cancer Treatments
www.paactusa.org
Prostate Cancer Education Council
www.pcaw.com
Prostate Cancer Foundation
www.pcf.org
Prostate Cancer Research and Education Foundation
www.pcref.org
Prostate Cancer Research Institute
www.prostate-cancer.org
Prostate Forum
www.prostateforum.com
The Prostate Net
www.prostate-online.org
Us TOO International Prostate Cancer Education and
Support Network
www.ustoo.org
Zero—The Project to End Prostate Cancer
www.zerocancer.org

Other Titles by Dr. Mark Moyad

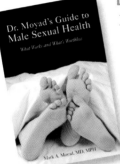

Dr. Moyad's Guide to Male Sexual Health

Dr. Moyad takes a candid look at all the topics that men and their partners have wondered about and answers the questions that they have been afraid to ask.

ISBN: 978-1-938170-01-0

Price: $15.95

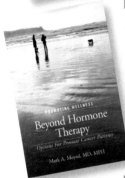

Promoting Wellness Beyond Hormone Therapy

Answering questions for patients whose prostate cancer is considered "hormone-refractory," this book provides a wealth of valuable resources for patients, caregivers, and health-care professionals alike.

ISBN: 978-1-58726-682-9

Price: $19.95

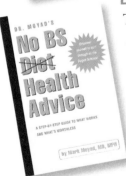

Dr. Moyad's No BS Health Advice

Taking a common sense and often light-hearted approach, Dr. Moyad pulls back the curtain on many half-truths and helps you develop a plan to improve your immune health and wellness.

ISBN: 978-1-58726-256-2

Price: $19.95

For more information please visit us online at:

www.sprypub.com

or contact us: Phone: 877-722-2264 Email: info@sprypub.com

Index